Final MB

A GUIDE TO SUCCESS IN CLINICAL MEDICINE

This book is dedicated to our partners Helen, Jo, Melanie and Jane

Commissioning Editor: Laurence Hunter
Project Development Manager: Janice Urquhart
Design Direction: Erik Bigland
Project Manager: Frances Affleck
Illustration Manager: Bruce Hogarth

Final MB

A GUIDE TO SUCCESS IN CLINICAL MEDICINE

H. R. Dalton BSc DPhil (Oxon) FRCP DipMedEd
Consultant Physician, Royal Cornwall Hospital, Truro, Cornwall, UK

N. J. Reynolds BSc MD FRCP
Professor of Dermatology, University of Newcastle-upon-Tyne, UK

S. I. R. Noble MB BS MRCP PGCE DipPalMed
Senior Lecturer in Palliative Medicine, Cardiff University Medical
School, Cardiff, UK

D. P. B. McGovern MB BS MRCP
Specialist Registrar in Gastroenterology, Oxford, UK

FOURTH EDITION

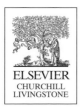

ELSEVIER
CHURCHILL
LIVINGSTONE

EDINBURGH LONDON NEW YORK OXFORD PHILADELPHIA
ST LOUIS SYDNEY TORONTO 2005

ELSEVIER
CHURCHILL
LIVINGSTONE

© Elsevier Limited 2001, 2003, 2005. All rights reserved.

The right of H. R. Dalton, N. J. Reynolds, S. I. R. Noble, and D. P. B. McGovern to be identified as authors of this work has been asserted by them in accordance with the Copyright, Designs and Patents Act 1988

First edition 1991
Second edition 1997
Third edition 2001
Fourth edition 2005
  Reprinted 2008

ISBN 978 0443 10049 9

British Library Cataloguing in Publication Data
A catalogue record for this book is available from the British Library

Library of Congress Cataloging in Publication Data
A catalog record for this book is available from the Library of Congress

Note
Medical knowledge is constantly changing. Standard safety precautions must be followed, but as new research and clinical experience broaden our knowledge, changes in treatment and drug therapy may become necessary or appropriate. Readers are advised to check the most current product information provided by the manufacturer of each drug to be administered to verify the recommended dose, the method and duration of administration, and contraindications. It is the responsibility of the practitioner, relying on experience and knowledge of the patient, to determine dosages and the best treatment for each individual patient. Neither the Publisher nor the authors assume any liability for any injury and/or damage to persons or property arising from this publication.

your source for books,
journals and multimedia
in the health sciences
www.elsevierhealth.com

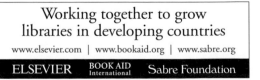

Working together to grow
libraries in developing countries

www.elsevier.com | www.bookaid.org | www.sabre.org

ELSEVIER   BOOK AID International   Sabre Foundation

The publisher's policy is to use paper manufactured from sustainable forests

Printed in China

Preface

Most medical schools worldwide now examine for the Final MB by an Objective Structured Clinical Examination (OSCE) in one form or another. This fourth edition of *Final MB*, together with its new companion text *Communication Skills for Final MB*, has been written to reflect these changes. We hope that these texts will enable the student to approach the Final Examination with confidence.

Both texts emphasise the basic principles required to approach the examination, followed by the most frequently occurring examination questions. We have been unable to cover all possible questions that you may face, but we hope that an understanding of the basic principles outlined in these books will give you the tools to approach any scenario successfully.

Final MB concentrates on practical examination subjects such as clinical examination, ECGs, radiographs and death certification. New sections on interpreting blood test results and on ethics have been included in this edition, following feedback from students.

At the ends of some of the chapters there are 'key questions' sections. These consist of samples of questions which are among the more frequently asked, and are included for you to consider. You will find many, but not all, of the answers in the main text. If you can't find the answer, discuss it with your colleagues or look it up in one of those big fat reference books.

Cornwall
2005

H.R.D.
N.J.R.
S.I.R.N.
D.P.B.McG.

Acknowledgements

We would like to thank Laurence Hunter and Janice Urquhart of Elsevier for their continued encouragement and support. We would also like to thank Dr Victoria Wheatley and Dr Melanie Jefferson for their help with the Ethics section.

Contents

PART 1

GENERAL PRINCIPLES

An overview of the examination

In recent years the final MB examination has changed in a major way: it has been restructured to ensure that the student is examined in as objective a manner as possible, which entails students being tested on similar or identical subjects.

The examination involves stations of a practical nature, which are discussed in this book. There is, however, a major emphasis on communication skills. The approach to this important topic is covered in the depth it deserves in our companion text *Communication Skills for Final MB*.

The subject matter of the Final MB examination has also changed: it now much more closely reflects the skills and competencies that you will need on your first day as a doctor. For example, it is now common to be asked to perform Basic Life Support and interpret ECGs, radiographs or blood test results. This seems to us an entirely appropriate change in the emphasis of the content of the examination.

The examination is marked by an objective tick box method (see Part 2), which makes it boring for the examiners. It also makes it an examination in which it is quite hard to excel; however, there are a number of basic things you can do to increase the chances of passing:

- Approach each question in a thorough and rigorous fashion.
- Appreciate what the examiners are looking for.
- Make sure you get a mark in each tick box.
- Project a professional demeanour and appearance.

Equipment

MIND AND BODY

The most important piece of equipment is yourself: your mind and body must be sharp and in good working order on the big day. It is up to you to make sure that this is the case. Do not stay up all night before the day of the examination learning the 25 causes of atrial fibrillation, as you will be in no fit state to remember them in the high-pressure setting of the examination room. Get an early night if you can. A tot of whisky may help you sleep. We do not recommend any other kind of hypnotic.

A few candidates go to extreme lengths during the run-up to the examinations. Some stay up all night trying to cram in those extra facts, filling themselves with endless cups of strong coffee. This is not recommended. Try to appreciate the difference between the time spent revising when you are alert and when you are not. A good hour's work when your mind is sharp is worth at least three when you are overtired with caffeine toxicity.

One or two candidates get so wound up by feelings of impending doom that they resort to pharmacological manipulations to try to improve their performance during the revision period, or during the examination itself. We cannot stress how important it is to avoid this. It is a recipe for disaster. If you are in this position you ought to go and see someone you trust (preferably a doctor), *now*. Drugs which have been used are caffeine-based stimulants (to keep awake to revise), hypnotics (to sleep after a hard day's revising) and beta-blockers (to keep calm).

All of the above drugs have central nervous system effects and will impair your mental agility on the day. Do not take them. A couple of drinks at 10.30 p.m. in the local pub with colleagues after a hard day's revision is much kinder on the central nervous system, and infinitely more pleasant.

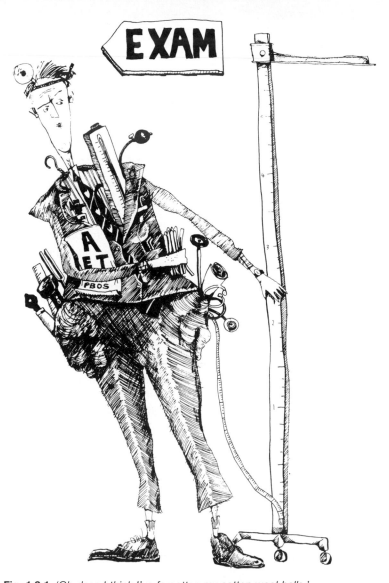

Fig. 1.2.1 *'Oh dear, I think I've forgotten my cotton wool balls.'*

EQUIPMENT TO TAKE WITH YOU

Stethoscope

You should take your own stethoscope with you. You need to check that it works properly before the exam. A contemporary of ours had the earpieces of his stethoscope blocked up as a practical joke (by so-called 'friends') prior to his clinical finals! He could not hear a thing through it during the exam, but luckily he still managed to pass.

Ophthalmoscope

You ought to take your own, for several reasons. If you have not got one don't worry — one will be provided. Ophthalmoscopes vary in design; it is important to get to know yours before the exam. Get to know which knobs do what, and make sure the batteries are new and the lenses are clean.

Neurological equipment

This will be provided at the examination. It is probably worth having some simple sensory testing equipment such as:

- *throw away* pins (HIV risk)
- cotton wool ball
- tape measure.

These will not take up much room in your pockets.

Tuning forks, patella hammers, smell bottles, Snellen charts, etc. are best left for the medical school to provide, as they are rather bulky items (Fig. 1.2.1).

PART 2

OSCEs: CLINICAL SKILLS

Note. Please note the following symbols which are used throughout this part of the book:

* — indicates cases that frequently crop up in the Final MB
† — indicates more complicated cases that occur only rarely.

2.1

General approach

The primary purpose of the clinical OSCEs is to objectively assess a student's clinical skills. In addition, in most clinical OSCEs marks will also be awarded for your attitude to the patient (and perhaps the examiner). Because of the way in which OSCEs are marked, it is very important to be methodical. What we mean by this is having a set routine for the examination of any organ system or part of the body which you may be asked to examine. In order to avoid getting poor marks, it is also crucial to have a methodical approach to the whole case (see later).

Structure

The Final MB OSCE examination varies from medical school to medical school in the time allocated to each OSCE station and the number of stations. However, a typical OSCE examination would be $2\frac{1}{2}$–3 hours long, have 10 to 12 stations of 7–10 minutes each, several rest stations and one or two larger stations of 20–30 minutes for history-taking, etc.

What is common to all OSCE examinations is that the same examiner examines all the students going through an individual OSCE station, using a standardised, objective marking sheet.

Content

The content of the OSCE stations largely covers three main areas:

- clinical examination skills (i.e. patients)
- practical skills
- communication skills.

This part of the book will concentrate on clinical examination skills. OSCEs covering practical skills are discussed in Part 3 (p. 151).

Some Final MB OSCE examinations include stations on paediatrics, psychiatry and surgery. This is beyond the scope of this book, and we would recommend you read the appropriate standard texts in these areas.

Marking

To make the assessment of students objective, a structured tick box mark sheet is used by the examiners. It is very important that you understand this, as you need to know on what criteria you are being assessed in order to get a good mark.

A typical OSCE mark sheet is shown in Table 2.1.1. The patient in question has aortic stenosis, which has caused him to be breathless due to left ventricular failure.

Consider two students, A and B. Student A is of below-average ability and is rather a 'plodder'. However, student A has a methodical approach to the case, introduces himself (1 mark) and has a good rapport with the patient and examiner (2 marks). Student A does a full and methodical examination of the cardiovascular system (7 marks), but diagnoses mitral incompetence as the cause of the patient's breathlessness, which is incorrect (0). The case is presented in a reasonable manner despite having the wrong diagnosis ($1\frac{1}{2}$ marks). The plan of investigation was correct (3 marks) as plans are identical for mitral incompetence and aortic stenosis (see Table 2.1.2).

Total marks, Student A: $14\frac{1}{2}$/20 — PASS.

Student B is mercurial, a quite brilliant student in the top 5% of the year. She is a high-flyer and always gets the diagnosis right. However, student B tends to be a bit slap-dash and in the heat of the examination setting forgets to introduce herself to the patient (0 marks) and is a bit abrupt with the patient ($\frac{1}{2}$ mark). Furthermore, she does not examine the peripheral pulses, BP, JVP, carotids and liver edge, but just listens to the precordium (3 marks). The findings are presented in a confident manner, but relevant positive findings (slow rising pulse, low BP) were not emphasised, as she did not examine them (2 marks). In the investigation plan she went straight for the echocardiograph and forgot the ECG and CXR (1 mark) (Table 2.1.2).

Total marks, Student B: $9\frac{1}{2}$/20 — FAIL!

Summary

Students A and B illustrate that the most important aspect of clinical skills OSCEs is not getting the diagnosis right, but getting

Table 2.1.1 Typical OSCE tick box mark sheet

Q This patient has been breathless. Examine his cardiovascular system. What is the differential diagnosis and how would you investigate him?

		Total possible marks	Sub-totals
Introduction	Student introduces themselves to patient and asks permission	1	1
Attitude	Student has professional attitude to patient and examiner	2	2
Examination	• Peripheral pulses and peripheral oedema	1	7
	• BP	1	
	• JVP and carotids	1	
	• Precordium	2	
	• Lung bases	1	
	• Liver and aortic abdominal aneurysm	1	
Presentation	• Findings presented in articulate and logical manner	2	3
	• Positive and relevant negative findings appropriately emphasised	1	
Differential diagnosis	Accurate differential diagnosis:		4
	• Aortic stenosis	4	
	• Aortic sclerosis		
Investigations	Appropriate investigation in sequential order:		3
	• ECG	1	
	• CXR	1	
	• Echocardiograph	1	
	Total		20
	(pass mark = 10)		

marks in all the boxes by being methodical. In the pressure of the examination it is easy to forget to introduce yourself to the patient or just examine the heart when you should be examining the whole of the cardiovascular system. Probably the best way to address this issue is continued practice until you are on 'automatic pilot'.

Table 2.1.2 OSCE mark sheets of students A and B		
	Student A	*Student B*
Introduction	1	0
Attitude	2	$\frac{1}{2}$
Examination	7	3
Presentation	$1\frac{1}{2}$	2
Differential diagnosis	0	3
Investigations	3	1
Total	$14\frac{1}{2}$ (PASS)	$9\frac{1}{2}$ (FAIL)

The concept of being on 'automatic pilot' is a simple one. You need to practise your examination technique in a pressure setting, preferably with a senior doctor watching. Practise examining any system, organ or anatomical region you can think of. Practise it again and again (under pressure). Eventually you will achieve the dizzy heights of being on 'automatic pilot'. That is, you will not need to think about what bit to examine next (when you are asked to examine a cardiovascular system for example) because you will do it automatically. You are now free to think about other things during the examination, such as making it look stylish and professional, identifying the physical signs and determining the differential diagnosis and the most appropriate plan of investigation.

Most OSCE stations should allow sufficient time for students to gather their thoughts before presenting their findings. Make sure you use this time to think about:

• signs you have elicited
• differential diagnosis
• plan of investigation.

Most students find it useful to time themselves doing a mock OSCE before the real thing. It takes most students approximately 5 minutes to do a thorough methodical examination of the cardiovascular system.

The rest of this section of the book (Chapters 2.2–2.10) deals with the types of questions you are likely to be asked, and the types of patients you are likely to meet during your clinical skills OSCE exam. We have emphasised the cases which frequently crop up in the Final MB clinical examination, and these are denoted by the symbol '*' in the text. We have also briefly mentioned the rarer, more complicated cases which appear occasionally: these are denoted by the symbol '†'. Some UK medical schools have OSCE 'death stations'. What this means is that if you fail one (or sometimes two) of these you fail the whole examination outright (p. 245). These are denoted by the symbol.

2.2

The cardiovascular system (CVS)

You will be asked to do one of five things. Do exactly what the examiner asks you to.

(i) Examine the CVS

This implies a full examination of the CVS. The patient should be comfortable on pillows at 45°. Introduce yourself and ask the patient if you may proceed with the examination. You should start at the hands and work your way up the arms to the face. Then examine the carotid pulse and JVP and then the heart. Do not forget to listen to the lung bases, feel for a liver edge, and abdominal aortic aneurysm. Feel all the peripheral pulses and for peripheral oedema. Do not forget to listen for bruits (including renal artery) and to feel for radiofemoral delay.

Follow the scheme set out in Table 2.2.1.

(ii) Examine the heart

You should do exactly the same as in (i), starting at the hands. The examiner may stop you and tell you just to listen to the heart, but at least you have demonstrated that you are aware that the examination of the heart starts at the hands.

(iii) Auscultate the heart

Do exactly what you have been told. Forget the hands and peripheral stuff and get your stethoscope plugged in.

Table 2.2.1 Scheme for examination of the CVS

General inspection
Hands
- peripheral cyanosis
- pallor
- clubbing (cyanotic congenital heart disease)
- splinters (infective endocarditis)
- nailfold infarction
- Quincke's sign (capillary pulsation of the nail beds found in aortic incompetence)

Radial pulse (make sure you time it with the second hand of your watch and examine both pulses)
- rate
- rhythm
- character

Radiofemoral delay — coarctation of aorta
Blood pressure
Conjunctivae — anaemia
Mouth — mucosal membranes, central cyanosis or pallor
Carotid pulses (both) — but not at the same time

JVP
Make sure you examine the *internal* jugular vein. The patient's neck must be relaxed. Remember the hepatojugular reflex. If you can't see the top of the JVP, sit the patient up to 90°. Earlobes will waggle if the JVP is very high

Look at the precordium
Scars (previous surgery)
Visible pulsations

Apex beat
Position: you must be seen to assess the exact position in terms of its relationship to the intercostal space (from the angle of Louis) and the mid-clavicular line
Quality:
- diffuse (LV dilatation)
- thrusting (LV hypertrophy)
- dyskinetic segment (LV aneurysm)

Palpate precordium
Thrills (palpable murmurs): this is best done over each valvular area with the palm of the hand. The metacarpal heads seem to be the most sensitive area of the hand to use for this
Palpable heart sounds: for all intents and purposes this means feel for the first heart sound of mitral stenosis, which is frequently palpable. It is this which gives the apex beat its 'tapping' quality in this condition (difficult sign)

Auscultation
Murmurs
Third and fourth heart sounds

Table 2.2.1 (*continued*)

Listen over each valvular area in turn with both the bell and diaphragm. Do not forget to turn the patient into the left lateral position and listen to the apex and axilla for mitral murmurs. Always sit the patient forwards and listen in expiration to the aortic area and down the left sternal edge for the murmur of aortic incompetence. While in this position, listen for carotid radiation/carotid bruits

Both bases
The patient is now sitting up. Take the opportunity to listen to both lung bases for crackles (left ventricular failure)

Abdomen
Liver, pulsatile (tricuspid regurgitation)
Abdominal aortic aneurysm
Renal artery bruits

Legs
Peripheral pulses — examine all of them
Peripheral oedema

(iv) Examine the pulse

You will usually be offered the right radial. If it is difficult to feel, go to the left radial or carotid. Time the pulse with the second hand of your watch. When examining the carotid pulse, do the right carotid artery with the left thumb and the left carotid artery with the right thumb.

The following parameters must be assessed when examining a pulse:

- rate
- rhythm
- character
  - slow rising (aortic stenosis)
  - water hammer (aortic regurgitation)
  - bisferiens (the double-topped pulse found in mixed aortic valve disease).

Occasionally the carotid pulse is visible from the end of the bed in aortic regurgitation (Corrigan's sign). In very severe aortic regurgitation the head may actually nod. This is called De Musset's sign.

(v) Examine the JVP

The patient must be at 45° with the head tilted and supported by a pillow to relax the strap muscles of the neck. It is usually best to turn the patient's face towards the left to achieve this. The JVP is best assessed in natural light; this may not be possible in the examination setting. It is essential to assess the internal jugular vein, not the external jugular. The external jugular vein may be raised due to local entrapment in the neck as it passes through the strap muscles and must therefore not be used as an indicator of the central venous pressure.

You need to know how to differentiate the JVP from carotid pulsation. The features to look for are:

- Double impulse in venous pulsation (not present in atrial fibrillation).
- The JVP falls on sitting up (usually). Carotid pulsation will not.
- Hepatojugular reflex. Venous return to the heart can be increased by pressing on the liver area. This will cause pulsation in the neck due to the JVP becoming more prominent. This distinguishes it from carotid pulsation.
- Filling from above. The JVP will fill from above when the internal jugular vein is pressed on firmly. Carotid pulsation will not.
- JVP is usually impalpable; carotid pulsation is usually palpable.
- Level of pulsation in JVP usually falls in inspiration.

A raised JVP may be found in many conditions, but the common ones found in the examination are:

- Severe right ventricular failure with tricuspid regurgitation; this may be secondary to valvular heart disease, ischaemic heart disease, cor pulmonale or cardiomyopathy.
- Fluid overload.

TYPICAL CASES

CVS

- Common murmurs
- Right-sided murmurs
- Ventricular septal defect
- Atrial septal defect

- Ischaemic heart disease
- Atrial fibrillation
- Left ventricular failure
- Hypertension
- Coarctation of the aorta
- Situs inversus/dextrocardia
- Aortic aneurysm

Cardiovascular cases are common in Final MB. This is because valvular heart disease is common (although now becoming less so) and the signs are chronic.

Common murmurs* (see Table 2.2.2)

Ischaemic heart disease

Common long case (angina or post-myocardial infarction). Uncommon short case. History is very important:

- cardiac pain
- past medical history of hypertension, diabetes or hyperlipidaemia
- family history
- smoking.

Signs

The patient may have no signs, but look for xanthelasmata, hypertension, signs of diabetes, signs of left ventricular dysfunction. The ECG may be normal.

Atrial fibrillation*

Very common Final MB case.

Signs

Irregularly irregular pulse. No 'a' waves in JVP (distinguishes it from multiple ventricular ectopics, which can also cause an irregularly irregular pulse). ECG shows irregular QRS complex with no 'P' waves (see p. 173).

Table 2.2.2 Common Final MB murmurs

Murmur	Sign	Associated findings	Causes
Aortic stenosis	Ejection systolic murmur which radiates to carotids	Slow rising pulse Heaving apex Low systolic BP LVH on ECG and CXR	Congenital (bifid valve) Rheumatic
Aortic incompetence (regurgitation)	Blowing early diastolic murmur (aortic area or LSE with patient sitting up in expiration)	Water-hammer pulse Wide pulse pressure Corrigan's sign De Musset's sign Quincke's sign Heaving apex LVH on ECG and CXR	Rheumatic Dissecting aortic aneurysm Ankylosing spondylitis Marfan's syndrome Congenital Syphilis
Mitral stenosis	Rumbling mid-diastolic murmur at apex	Palpable first heart sound Presystolic accentuation if patient in sinus rhythm AF Opening snap	Usually rheumatic
Mitral incompetence	Pansystolic murmur at apex	Radiates to axilla, best heard left lateral position	Rheumatic LV dilatation (any cause) Ruptured chordae, etc.

Note. *Aortic sclerosis* has exactly the same murmur as *aortic stenosis*, but none of the associated physical findings. It is due to thickening of the aortic valve (calcific age-related change) and is of no clinical significance, except that it has to be distinguished from aortic stenosis.

Causes

- Ischaemic heart disease*
- Post-myocardial infarction*
- Mitral stenosis*
- Thyrotoxicosis
- Pulmonary embolism
- ASD
- Hypertensive heart disease
- Malignant infiltration of pericardium.

Left ventricular failure

Although this is a very common diagnosis in everyday clinical practice, it is not often included in the examination. The reason for this is that patients with acute left ventricular failure are too unwell to be included. You may get someone in the recovery phase, but by this stage the signs will be disappearing or have gone altogether.

Signs

- Tachypnoea
- Central cyanosis
- Sinus tachycardia
- Third heart sound
- Crackles at both bases.

ECG shows left ventricular strain pattern. CXR shows cardiomegaly, upper lobe blood diversion, interstitial shadowing, Kerley B lines, bat's wing appearance (see p. 204).

Hypertension

Ninety per cent of the cases are primary*. Ten per cent are secondary to:

- renal disease*
- coarctation of the aorta
- Cushing's disease
- Conn's syndrome
- acromegaly
- phaeochromocytoma.

Signs

Look for the effects of hypertension on the:

- Eyes
    - a-v nipping
    - increased vessel tortuosity
    - haemorrhage
    - exudates
    - papilloedema
- Heart — signs of LVH, ischaemic heart disease
- Kidneys — signs of chronic renal failure
- Peripheral vasculature.

You need to know a little bit about the investigations and the treatment of hypertension. These are commonly asked questions.

Right-sided murmurs[†]

- Tricuspid regurgitation
- Pulmonary stenosis
- Pulmonary incompetence
- Tricuspid stenosis.

Most examiners regard these as postgraduate murmurs.

Ventricular septal defect (VSD)[†]

Rare. Sounds like mitral regurgitation at the left sternal edge (pansystolic, harsh).

Causes

- Congenital (maladie de Roger)
- Post-MI (septal rupture — you will not see this in an exam as the patients are too sick).

Atrial septal defect (ASD)[†]

Rare. Fixed splitting of second heart sound with a pulmonary systolic flow murmur (postgraduate murmur).

Cause

- Congenital.

Coarctation of the aorta[†]

This is a very rare cause of hypertension.

Signs

- Radiofemoral delay.
- You can sometimes hear odd murmurs on the upper chest and back due to blood flow through the collaterals.
- Hypertension in the arms, hypotension in the legs.
- CXR (see p. 207)
  - rib notching
  - post-stenotic dilatation of aorta.

Situs inversus/dextrocardia[†]

This is very very rare, but much loved by the examiners.

Causes

Dextrocardia is one of the few causes of inaudible heart sounds. Other causes are:

- obesity*
- chronic obstructive airways disease*
- left pleural effusion (large)
- pericardial effusion
- stethoscope not adjusted properly*.

If you think your patient has dextrocardia, other organs could also be transposed. There is an association with Kartagener's syndrome.

Aortic aneurysm

- Abdominal — this is really a surgical case.
- Thoracic[†] — the patient will complain of back and chest pain or a hoarse voice; signs include a tracheal tug and aortic regurgitation.

Causes

- Syphilis
- Atheroma
- Post-dissection of aorta
- Traumatic.

KEY QUESTIONS

CVS

1. **What are the causes of:**
   - atrial fibrillation
   - sinus tachycardia
   - sinus bradycardia
   - a raised JVP
   - aortic regurgitation
   - aortic stenosis
   - mitral regurgitation
   - mitral stenosis
   - left ventricular failure
   - an impalpable apex
   - hypertension?
2. **What are the risk factors associated with ischaemic heart disease?**
3. **How can you tell the difference clinically between:**
   - a raised JVP and a visible carotid pulsation
   - the murmur of aortic regurgitation and mitral stenosis
   - the murmur of mitral regurgitation and aortic stenosis
   - aortic stenosis and aortic sclerosis?

2.3

The respiratory system

The standard question asked is: 'Examine this patient's chest/ respiratory system'. This should be done quickly but professionally. The patient should be comfortable, propped up by pillows at 45°. Introduce yourself. Ask permission to examine the patient. The guide for examination of the respiratory system is set out in Table 2.3.1.

TYPICAL CASES

The respiratory system

- Clubbing
- Carcinoma of lung
- Chronic obstructive airways disease
- Asthma
- Pleural effusion
- Fibrosing alveolitis
- Pneumothorax
- Sarcoidosis
- Haemoptysis
- Thoracoplasty/physical treatments for TB
- Superior vena cava obstruction
- Cor pulmonale
- Pneumonia
- Bronchiectasis

Clubbing*

Very common case.

Causes

- Carcinoma of the bronchus*
- Chronic suppurative lung disease
- mesothelioma

Table 2.3.1

General inspection
Respiratory rate
Hands
- clubbing (bronchial carcinoma)
- nicotine staining (COAD, bronchial carcinoma)
- CO_2 retention flap (respiratory failure)
- essential tremor (β_2 agonist therapy)
- peripheral cyanosis

Pulse
Conjunctivae — suffusion (polycythaemia in COAD, or SVC obstruction)
Anaemia
Mucosae of mouth — central cyanosis
Trachea position — think of things which push (pleural effusion) or pull (collapse) to one side
Nodes
- supraclavicular
- cervical
- occipital
- axillary

  Supraclavicular nodes are best felt from behind to allow the fingertips to get right in behind the clavicles

JVP
Raised in cor pulmonale and SVC obstruction

Apex beat
Determine the position exactly. This will, together with the tracheal position, allow you to determine if there is any mediastinal shift. If the apex beat is impalpable, this is also useful information, e.g. COAD

Right ventricular heave
Cor pulmonale

Expansion
This is arguably the most important sign in chest medicine. It is done quite badly and is quite tricky to do well. Get an experienced doctor to show you how. It tells you where the pathology is (pathology = side with least expansion). It is bilaterally decreased in COAD

Percussion
Auscultation   } Compare right with
Tactile vocal fremitus   left on front of
Auditory resonance   } chest

  Now you need to sit the patient forward and repeat the above examination from 'expansion' on the back of the chest

---

Table 2.3.1 (continued)
Whispering pectoriloquy This is an over-rated clinical sign. The way to elicit it is to get the patient to whisper 'one, one, one'. The sounds are heard better over an area of consolidation or the top of a pleural effusion
Examine the ankles for pitting oedema (cor pulmonale?)
Sputum pot Do not forget to look for it. It may give an important clue to the diagnosis, e.g. haemoptysis
CXR Ask to see it

- — cystic fibrosis
- — empyema
- — bronchiectasis
- — lung abscess
- Fibrosing alveolitis
- Congenital cyanotic heart disease
- Familial
- Idiopathic
- Infective endocarditis[†]   ○ atrial myxoma
- Cirrhosis of liver[†]
- Ulcerative colitis[†]
- Crohn's disease[†].
- Coeliac

None c̄: COPD
EAA
Sarcoid

You *must* know this list.

Carcinoma of lung*

Very common case.

Signs

Look for:

- cachexia
- clubbing
- nicotine-stained fingers
- lymph nodes

- signs of intrathoracic involvement, e.g.:
  — pleural effusion
  — collapse
  — recurrent chest infections.

Ask to see the chest X-ray and sputum pot.

Remember Pancoast's tumour. This is a carcinoma of the bronchus at the apex causing an ipsilateral Horner's syndrome (involvement of sympathetic chain) and ipsilateral wasting of the small muscles of the hand (T1 root of brachial plexus involved).

Chronic obstructive airways disease*

Common case.

Signs

- Nicotine-stained fingers
- CO_2 retention flap (rare in the exam)
- β_2 agonist tremor
- Tachypnoea
- Pursed lip breathing   } 'pink puffer'
- Using accessory muscles of respiration
- Centrally cyanosed   } 'blue bloater'
- Peripheral oedema
- Overexpansion/barrel-shaped chest
- Hyperresonant percussion note
- Loss of cardiac dullness
- Impalpable apex beat
- Distant heart sounds
- Wheeze/reduced air entry.

You need to know about the aetiology, treatment and chest X-ray appearance. Patients have an obstructive deficit on respiratory function testing with an FEV_1/FVC ratio of less than 0.75.

Asthma

Acute asthma will not appear in the examination for obvious reasons. A patient in the recovery phase from an acute attack or a patient with the more chronic variety is sometimes included.

Signs

There may be none. The patient may be overexpanded or there may be wheeze in the chest. Ask to look at the peak flow chart.

From Figure 2.3.1 you ought to note that the patient has morning dips and that there is a gradual increase in the peak flow as the patient recovers. In addition to this there is also a gradual reduction in the diurnal variation in peak flow as the patient recovers. Figure 2.3.2 shows a peak flow recorded in chronic asthma. Again note the morning dips around the average of 300 l/min.

Pleural effusion

This will usually crop up if there happens to be a patient with a pleural effusion on the ward at the time of the exam. Chronic pleural effusion in out-patients is uncommon.

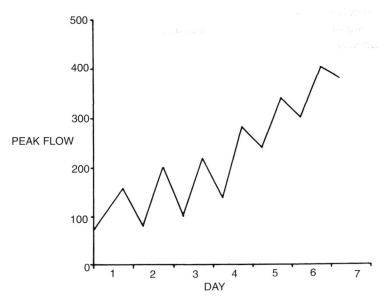

Fig. 2.3.1 Peak expiratory flow rate of recovery from acute severe asthma. Note that the morning 'dipping' improves as the patient recovers.

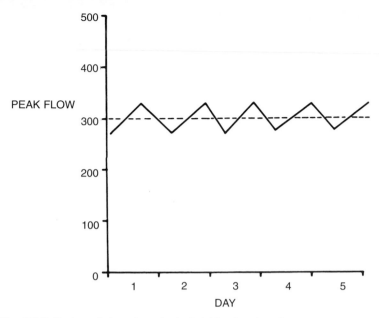

Fig. 2.3.2 Peak expiratory flow chart of stable chronic asthma.

Signs

- Reduced expansion
- Stony, dull percussion note
- Absent breath sounds
- There may be bronchial breathing and/or whispering pectoriloquy over the top of the effusion
- Mediastinum may be shifted away from the side of the effusion, if it is a large one
- Signs of previous pleural tap, e.g. sticking plaster on patient's back.

Causes

1. Exudate — protein content greater than 30 g/l
2. Transudate — protein content less than 30 g/l.

   Exudate

- Neoplastic
  — secondary pleural deposits, e.g. from lung or breast*
  — primary mesothelioma

- Inflammatory — following pneumonia*
  - bacterial
  - viral
  - tuberculosis
- Pulmonary embolus
- Trauma
- Rheumatoid arthritis, SLE
- Subphrenic abscess, pancreatitis.

Transudate

- Heart failure*
- Cirrhosis of liver*
- Nephrotic syndrome
- Meigs' syndrome.

Fibrosing alveolitis

Although this condition is not that common, the signs are chronic and such patients are frequently included.

Signs

- Clubbing
- Central cyanosis
- Reduced expansion (bilateral)
- Bilateral fine inspiratory crackles, worse at bases.

Causes

- Idiopathic*
- Rheumatoid arthritis
- SLE
- Asbestosis.

The idiopathic variety often responds to steroids, so look for the Cushingoid appearance and easy bruising.

Chest X-ray shows reduced lung volumes and fluffy shadows, which start at the bases and work upwards. They make the heart border and diaphragm indistinct.

Respiratory function shows a restrictive deficit with FEV_1/FVC greater than 75% and the transfer factor and vital capacity will invariably be reduced.

Pneumothorax[†]

This is a very rare exam case.

Sarcoidosis[†]

Rare Final MB case.

Signs

- Erythema nodosum
- Bilateral hilar lymphadenopathy on chest X-ray
- Bilateral uveitis
- Chest examination is often normal.

It can also cause (rarely) hepatomegaly, splenomegaly, skin deposits, VII nerve palsies (sometimes bilateral), diffuse CNS involvement. There is often a restrictive defect on the respiratory function tests with an FEV_1/FVC greater than 75% and a reduced transfer factor. If the patient is asymptomatic, no treatment is indicated. If symptomatic, or there is widespread disease or worsening transfer factor/X-ray, the patient should be treated with prednisolone.

Haemoptysis

You will occasionally be asked: 'Examine this patient who has been coughing up blood'. More commonly you will find blood in the sputum pot (if you remember to look in it) during the course of your examination.

Causes

Think of the following causes:

- pneumonia (bacterial)*
- carcinoma of the lung*
- tuberculosis*
- bronchiectasis
- post-traumatic
- pulmonary embolus
- mitral stenosis
- idiopathic (this is a common cause in young people in everyday practice, but not in the exam).

Thoracoplasty/physical treatments for TB[†]

Patients treated for tuberculosis up until the early 1950s used to have quite drastic surgical procedures as part of their management. They are becoming increasingly scarce as this cohort of patients ages. They are sometimes brought up for the exam.

Signs

- Thoracoplasty
- Ping pong balls — inserted into upper pleural space to maintain an artificial pneumothorax.

Superior vena cava obstruction[†]

This is rare as an examination case, but you need to look for plethora of the upper half of the body and conjunctival suffusion, fixed raised JVP, swelling of the arms, face and neck, and collateral vessels. The usual cause is carcinoma of the bronchus impinging on the superior vena cava. It can be treated radiologically by deploying a metal stent, or by radiotherapy. Look for marks on the chest to see if the patient has had or is having a course of radiotherapy.

Cor pulmonale

Students often get confused about this. Any chest condition causing prolonged hypoxia will eventually cause pulmonary hypertension. This is due to a direct effect of hypoxia on the pulmonary microcirculation. The pulmonary hypertension, in turn, causes a strain on the right side of the heart. This results in right ventricular hypertrophy and, eventually, right ventricular failure.

Signs

- Central cyanosis
- Right ventricular heave (felt with the flat of the hand at the left sternal edge)
- Raised JVP
- Peripheral oedema (pitting)
- There may also be hepatomegaly (pulsatile).

You need to remember to look for the causes of the cor pulmonale, e.g. chronic obstructive airways disease or fibrosing alveolitis.

Pneumonia

Cases of pneumonia in the final MB are uncommon. However, you may get a patient in the recovery phase.

Signs

You will need to look for signs of consolidation/collapse when examining the chest. The patient may have residual fever.

Causes

There are many causes of pneumonia but remember the following headings:

- Bacterial, e.g. *Streptococcus pneumoniae*, *Haemophilus influenzae*, tuberculosis, *Klebsiella*, *Staphylococcus*.
- Viral, including cytomegalovirus, influenza virus, RSV, adenovirus, etc.
- Rare causes, such as *Pneumocystis carinii*, yeasts and fungi (immunocompromised patient).

   Mycoplasma can cause pneumonia in otherwise fit adults.

Bronchiectasis

Signs

- Clubbing of fingernails
- Late inspiratory crackles (often unilateral).

   Sputum pot will show purulent, thick secretions and may also contain blood. The pathogenesis involves local dilatation of the bronchi with subsequent collection of purulent secretions.

Causes

- Tuberculosis
- Measles
- Post-nasal drip
- Foreign body
- Post-pneumonia
- Cystic fibrosis
- Idiopathic.

Table 2.3.2 Signs in respiratory disease. You may find the following table helpful in sorting out what is going on inside the chest when you are examining it

	Mediastinum	Expansion	Percussion note	Breath sounds	Tactile vocal fremitus
Pleural effusion	Moves away from affected side	↓	Stony dull	Absent	↓
Pneumothorax	No difference (away from affected side if tension)	↓	Hyperresonant	Absent	↓
Collapse	Towards affected side	↓	↓	↓ or ↑ if associated consolidation	↓
Consolidation	No change Towards affected side if associated collapse	↓	↓	↑ or bronchial breathing/whispering pectoriloquy	↑

Note. (1) Collapse and consolidation often coexist in real life, and so the signs are mixed.
(2) Bronchial breathing and whispering pectoriloquy can be heard above a pleural effusion (sometimes).

There is an association with Kartagener's syndrome. This is a combination of post-nasal drip, bronchiectasis and infertility. This is due to an abnormality of cilial function. Occasionally, situs inversus or dextrocardia is found in this syndrome.

KEY QUESTIONS

The respiratory system

1. **What are the causes of:**
   - clubbing of the finger nails
   - pleural effusion
   - haemoptysis
   - primary community-acquired chest infections
   - bronchiectasis
   - cor pulmonale?
2. **How would you differentiate clinically between:**
   - consolidation and collapse
   - pneumothorax and pleural effusion
   - peripheral and central cyanosis
   - restrictive and obstructive airways disease?
3. **Define central cyanosis.**
4. **What respiratory problems are encountered in patients with HIV-related disease?**

The gastrointestinal tract (GIT)

The GIT should be examined in a thorough, systematic way. It is important not to hurt the patient, and before you start your examination you should always ask if the patient has any tenderness in the abdomen. During the course of the examination it is essential to keep glancing at the patient's face, to ensure that you are not causing any discomfort. The other advantage of asking the patient if there is any pain or tenderness in the abdomen is that, if there is, the location of this tenderness may give an important clue as to the site of the pathology. For example, if the patient complains of tenderness in the right upper quadrant, the chances are that there is tender hepatomegaly.

The usual question asked in the Final MB is either to examine the GIT or examine the abdomen. This essentially means a full examination of the GIT, starting at the hands, as set out in Table 2.4.1. Occasionally you will be asked just to 'palpate the abdomen'. In this case, do exactly what you are told, and no more. However, do not forget to use your eyes, e.g. if you see a fullness in the left hypochondrium, make sure you feel particularly thoroughly for a spleen.

The patient should be laid flat in bed. If the patient is uncomfortable without a pillow, one should be provided. Traditionally the area from knees to nipples should be exposed, but in the exam setting the patient's modesty should be preserved, so the lower limit of exposure should be just above the pubis.

The general scheme for the examination of the GIT is set out in Table 2.4.1.

SPECIFIC POINTS TO NOTE ON GIT EXAMINATION

Observation of abdomen

Ask the patient to take a deep breath in while you observe the abdomen. This accentuates areas of fullness caused by underlying

Table 2.4.1 Scheme for examination of the GIT

General inspection
Wasting, scars, etc.

Hands
Clubbing (cirrhosis, Crohn's disease)
Palmar erythema, Dupuytren's contracture, leuconychia (chronic liver disease)

Liver flap
Hepatic encephalopathy

Conjunctivae
Jaundice, anaemia

Mouth
Telangiectasia (hereditary haemorrhagic telangiectasia)
Perioral pigmentation (Peutz-Jegher syndrome)

Tongue

Supraclavicular nodes
Virchow's node, Troisier's sign

Skin on chest wall
Spider naevi, gynaecomastia, bruising/purpura (chronic liver disease)

Observation of abdomen
Areas of fullness
• masses
• organomegaly
• ascites
Scars (see Fig. 2.4.1, p. 42)
Distended veins on the anterior abdominal wall. Determine direction of blood flow (see Fig. 2.4.2, p. 43)
Everted umbilicus (ascites; several litres of fluid needed to produce this sign)

Palpation
Light and deep, do each quadrant in turn
Feel for masses, organomegaly (liver, kidneys, spleen, bladder, uterus) and tenderness. Remember to look at the patient's face

Percussion
Areas of dullness corresponding to masses/organomegaly

Shifting dullness/fluid thrill

Auscultation
Bowel sounds — bruits (renal artery, aortic, hepatic)
'Liver scratch sign' (Fig. 2.4.3, p. 43)
Extra thinking time

Hernial orifices

Peripheral oedema

organomegaly/masses. Now ask the patient to raise the feet off the bed while you observe the abdomen. Any lurking incisional herniae or divarification of the recti will now be obvious.

Palpation

Palpation should be performed from the patient's right side while you are kneeling or sitting. The reason for this is that the hand is more relaxed and more in contact with the patient in this position. It is far more sensitive than examining the patient while you are in the standing position.

Liver

Start in the right iliac fossa (RIF) and work upwards, asking the patient to breathe in as you palpate.

Spleen

Start in the RIF and work towards the left hypochondrium. If you start in the left iliac fossa (LIF) or left hypochondrium you may miss a very large spleen. To feel a small spleen it may be necessary to get the patient to roll partly onto the right side and feel with the fingertips under the left costal margin (during inspiration). The spleen needs to be enlarged to at least twice its normal size for it to be palpable.

Percussion

Percuss the whole abdomen. Remember to percuss the upper border of the liver and spleen.

Ascites

Shifting dullness

Percuss out the anterior limit of the fluid level. This is best done with your finger parallel to the air–fluid interface (i.e. in the sagittal plane). Now ask the patient to roll onto the side. Re-percuss to assess if the area of dullness has moved, which indicates free fluid in the peritoneal space.

Fluid thrill

If you have demonstrated shifting dullness, go on to try to demonstrate a fluid thrill. Ask the examiner to place the hypothenar aspect of his hand firmly on the midline of the anterior abdominal wall (in the sagittal plane). Flick the fluid firmly on one side, while palpating the other.

Bruits

If you find hepatomegaly you must listen for a bruit over the liver. Liver bruits are rare and are caused by hepatoma, large hepatic haemangiomas and transjugular intrahepatic portosystemic shunts (TIPSS).

PR/genitals

Do not examine the genitals or perform a rectal examination, but express the desirability of doing so.

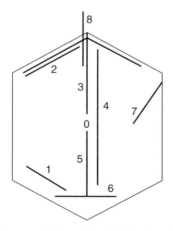

Fig. 2.4.1 Abdominal scars. 1 Appendix. 2 Cholecystectomy. 3 Gastric surgery. 4 Laparotomy. 5 Hysterectomy/Classical Caesarean. 6 Caesarean section. 7 Nephrectomy. 8. Liver transplant (Mercedes-Benz scar).

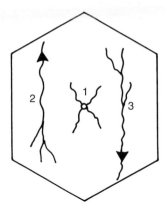

Fig. 2.4.2 Abnormal anterior abdominal veins. 1 *Caput medusae*; dilated veins around the umbilicus, found in portal hypertension: flow is away from the umbilicus. 2 *IVC obstruction*: flow upwards. 3 *SVC obstruction*: flow downwards.

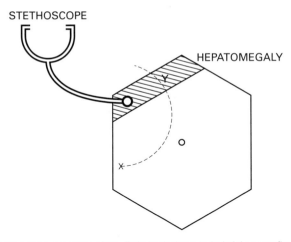

Fig. 2.4.3 The liver scratch sign. This technique is helpful to confirm the presence of hepatomegaly, suspected by palpation and percussion. It is particularly useful in the obese patient, when percussion and palpation of organs may be difficult. Listen with the stethoscope over the liver edge. At the same time lightly scratch the abdominal wall with the fingernail in the right iliac fossa (point X). Work your way upwards, scratching gently as you go but keeping your finger at the same distance from the stethoscope at all times. When you come over the liver edge (point Y), you will hear a loud scratching noise. This is because the scratching sound is being transmitted through the liver substance, which is solid and therefore a good sound conductor. Some older examiners don't like this sign.

TYPICAL CASES

GIT

- Hepatomegaly
- Splenomegaly
- Hepatosplenomegaly
- Ascites
- Mass in the abdomen
- Jaundice
- Anaemia
- Chronic liver disease.
- Carcinoid syndrome
- Polycystic liver disease
- Liver transplant
- Primary biliary cirrhosis
- Autoimmune chronic active hepatitis
- Crohn's disease
- Ulcerative colitis

Hepatomegaly*

Delineate the lower border of the liver, and size it in terms of finger breadths below the costal margin. Remember also to find where the upper border is (by percussion). This is important because occasionally a liver edge can be felt just below the costal margin when there is no true hepatomegaly, e.g. in chronic obstructive airways disease where hyperexpanded lungs push down the (normal-sized) liver.

Define the characteristics of the liver edge you have felt in terms of:

- the edge
  — smooth
  — knobbly (multiple metastases or cysts)
- pulsatility (tricuspid regurgitation)
- consistency
  — firm
  — hard
- bruit (hepatocellular carcinoma, a-v malformation, TIPSS)
- tenderness (hepatitis, capsular pain of the hepatomegaly of congestive cardiac failure).

Think of the causes of hepatomegaly and look for other signs which may give you the diagnosis of the patient in front of you (see Table 2.4.2).

Splenomegaly*

A favourite examiners' question is 'how can you tell the difference clinically between splenomegaly and a palpable left kidney?'

Table 2.4.2 Hepatomegaly: causes and signs to look for

Cause	Signs to look for
Chronic liver disease (of any aetiology)	See pp. 50–55
Fatty infiltration*	Usually no other signs
Metastatic carcinoma	Look for the site of primary • breasts • lung • prostate, etc.
Hepatitis[†] (A, B, C)	Jaundice, splenomegaly, tattoos, signs of i.v. drug abuse Ask about travel, transfusions, sexual history
Hepatoma[†]	Listen for bruit Ask about past history of hepatitis B or C, cirrhosis
Polycystic liver disease	Polycystic kidneys Signs of renal support (fistula)
Congestive cardiac failure (CCF)	↑ JVP Pulsatile liver Peripheral oedema
Lymphoma[†]	Splenomegaly, lymphadenopathy, fever, weight loss
Leukaemia (all types)[†]	Splenomegaly, nodes (CLL), purpura, petechiae, fever, etc.

Notes.
(1) In the later stages of cirrhosis the liver may be impalpable, as it is small, shrunken and fibrosed.
(2) Very rare exam cases: sarcoid; TB, infectious mononucleosis (EB virus, CMV, toxoplasmosis), RA, SLE.

Answer

The spleen has a notch, whereas a kidney does not. You can ballot a kidney but you cannot ballot a spleen. A spleen is dull to percussion, a kidney is not. You cannot get above a spleen, but you can sometimes get above a kidney.

Categories of splenomegaly

Splenomegaly is subjectively categorised as mild, moderate or large:

- Large (past umbilicus)
  — chronic granulocytic leukaemia
  — myelofibrosis
  — kala-azar[†] (*not* in UK).
- Moderate (up to the umbilicus)
  — lymphoma
  — chronic lymphatic leukaemia (CLL)
  — portal hypertension
  — malaria[†].
- Mild (just palpable)
  — portal hypertension (of any cause)
  — lymphoma
  — CLL
  — polycythaemia rubra vera
  — rheumatoid arthritis (ask to see full blood count result — Felty's syndrome)
  — SLE
  — amyloidosis   ⎫
  — hepatitis   ⎬ Rare in the exam.
  — infectious mononucleosis   ⎭
  — malaria

Hepatosplenomegaly*

Causes

- Chronic liver disease (of any cause) with portal hypertension*
- Lymphoma
- Leukaemia (any type)
- Infections[†]
  — hepatitis (A, B, C, CMV, EBV)
- Amyloid[†]

- Sarcoid[†]
- SLE.[†]

Ascites

You need to examine for this in the correct manner, as described earlier in the chapter. Fullness in both flanks on general inspection usually gives the game away (the only other common cause for this is polycystic disease of the kidneys). Look for an everted umbilicus.

Causes

The commonest cause, by far, is cirrhosis of the liver. It is helpful to think of the causes of ascites under the following headings:

- hypoalbuminaemia
  — chronic liver disease (any cause)*
  — protein-calorie malnutrition
  — nephrotic syndrome
  — protein-losing enteropathy
- portal hypertension — chronic liver disease*
- local inflammatory process
  — metastatic carcinoma (in the peritoneum)
  — pelvic carcinoma (ovary)
  — infection (e.g. peritoneal TB).

Mass in the abdomen

The patient can often help you, if you allow. Remember to ask if there is tenderness anywhere. If there is, ask where it is. This may well be of considerable help in localising the pathology. Think of the anatomical structures normally found in the area in which you have palpated the mass. This will help you to arrive at a reasonable differential diagnosis.

Causes

The causes of a mass in the abdomen depend on the location of the mass:

- RUQ
  — gallbladder
  — carcinoma head of pancreas

- — Reidel's lobe
- — right kidney
- — carcinoma colon (hepatic flexure)
- epigastrium
  - — carcinoma stomach
  - — enlarged left lobe liver
  - — pancreatic pseudocyst
  - — pancreatic carcinoma
  - — abdominal aortic aneurysm
- LUQ
  - — spleen
  - — left kidney
  - — carcinoma splenic flexure
  - — carcinoma tail of pancreas
- central/periumbilical
  - — abdominal aortic aneurysm
  - — carcinoma body of pancreas
  - — pancreatic pseudocyst
  - — lymphoma
- RIF
  - — carcinoma caecum
  - — right ovarian mass
  - — mass of matted small bowel (e.g. Crohn's)
- LIF
  - — carcinoma sigmoid colon
  - — left ovarian mass
  - — transplanted kidney.

Jaundice

The patient will almost invariably be an in-patient. This fact makes jaundice an uncommon examination case.

Causes

Remember the basic causes:

- Pre-hepatic
  - — autoimmune haemolytic anaemia
  - — drug-induced haemolytic anaemia (e.g. methyldopa)
  - — hereditary spherocytosis
  - — sickle cell anaemia

- thalassaemias
- transfusion reactions
- red cell fragmentation syndromes (e.g. DIC secondary to septicaemia)
- Gilbert's syndrome.
- Hepatic
  - chronic liver disease (any cause)
  - acute hepatitis (A, B, C, glandular fever, Weil's disease)
  - metastatic carcinoma of the liver
  - hepatotoxic drugs (e.g. post-paracetamol overdose, antibiotics such as Augmentin).
- Cholestasis
  - drugs, e.g. chlorpromazine
  - biliary obstruction
  - gallstones
  - carcinoma of pancreas
  - primary sclerosing cholangitis (PSC).

It can be difficult or impossible to distinguish between these causes clinically. Points to look out for which may give a clue are found in the patient's history, the examination, and the investigations (see below). The commonest causes are alcoholic hepatitis, cancer of the pancreas and metastatic liver disease. Pre-hepatic jaundice is very uncommon.

History

- Transfusions ⎫
- Travel
- Tattoos
- Drug abuse (intravenous) ⎬ Hepatitis B and C
- Sexual preferences
- Infectious contacts ⎭
- Job (sewers) — Weil's disease[†]
- Family history of jaundice or splenectomy (suggests haemolysis)
- Past history of recurrent jaundice
  - haemolysis
  - Gilbert's syndrome
- Drug history (see above)
- Alcohol intake
- Back/abdominal pains (pancreatitis/carcinoma of pancreas)
- Ulcerative colitis/fever/jaundice — PSC.

Examination

Look for:

- stigmata of chronic liver disease
- hepatomegaly (knobbly in secondary carcinoma)
- splenomegaly (haemolysis or portal hypertension)
- anaemia (haemolysis)
- palpable gallbladder (carcinoma of pancreas)
- needle puncture marks (hepatitis B and C).
  Patients with haemolytic jaundice have a lemon yellow tinge.

Investigations

- Raised unconjugated bilirubin
- Urobilinogen in urine
- Reduced haptoglobins

} Imply haemolytic jaundice.

Remember the Coombs' test, Hb electrophoresis and red cell fragility studies.

The ALT and AST are raised out of proportion to the alkaline phosphatase in hepatic jaundice.

Alkaline phosphatase is raised out of proportion to ALT in cholestasis. Ultrasound examination is essential to determine the calibre of the common bile duct. If this is dilated (>10 mm) it implies a surgical (cholestatic) cause for the jaundice.

Anaemia

This is unlikely to be the only sign. The causes are listed in Table 2.4.3.

Chronic liver disease*

This is a common short case, as chronic liver disease is common and it produces interesting, stable clinical signs. The clinical signs, complications and causes of chronic liver disease are shown in Table 2.4.4.

When you see a patient with signs suggestive of chronic liver disease, always check for signs of complications such as portal hypertension, hepatic encephalopathy or a primary liver cancer. It is usually not possible to make an accurate diagnosis as to the aetiology of the chronic liver disease from the clinical examination alone

---

Table 2.4.3 Causes of anaemia

Hypochromic microcytic
Iron deficiency due to:
Chronic blood loss
- peptic ulcer
- carcinoma of the stomach, colon or caecum
- colitis
- uterine
- renal tract
Malabsorption secondary to partial gastrectomy, extensive ileal resection, coeliac disease
Dietary
During pregnancy

Normochromic normocytic
Chronic disease
- rheumatoid arthritis
- systemic lupus erythematosus
- Crohn's disease
- carcinoma
- lymphoma
- chronic infections, e.g. TB

Macrocytic
B_{12} deficiency
- pernicious anaemia
- gastrectomy
- blind-loop syndrome
- tropical sprue
- ileal resection
- Crohn's disease
- dietary (veganism)
Folate deficiency
- dietary (alcoholics, old age, pregnancy)
- malabsorption (see above)
- increased utilisation of folate (pregnancy, haemolysis, myelosclerosis, carcinoma)
- anticonvulsant therapy

(a liver biopsy is usually required for this). However, there may be clues which suggest the diagnosis:

- i.v. puncture marks
  — hepatitis B, C
- middle-aged female with xanthelasmata
  — primary biliary cirrhosis (PBC)

Table 2.4.4 Signs, complications and causes of chronic liver disease

Signs
Palmar erythema, Dupuytren's
Spider naevi
Gynaecomastia
Testicular atrophy
Hepatomegaly
Ascites
Peripheral oedema
Jaundice
Muscle wasting
Clubbing of the fingernails[†]

Complications
Portal hypertension
• splenomegaly
• ascites
• abnormal abdominal veins
• oesophageal varices
Hepatic encephalopathy
• liver flap
• hepatic foetor
• mental obtundation
Gram-negative sepsis
Primary hepatocellular carcinoma (bruit over liver)

Causes
Common
• alcohol
• chronic hepatitis B, C
• autoimmune chronic active hepatitis
• primary biliary cirrhosis (PBC)
• cryptogenic
Uncommon
• primary sclerosing cholangitis (PSC)
• haemochromatosis
• α_1 antitrypsin deficiency
• Wilson's disease

• young female
   — autoimmune chronic active hepatitis
• ileostomy in a middle-aged male
   — primary sclerosing cholangitis (associated with ulcerative colitis)
• pigmentation
   — haemochromatosis

- Kayser–Fleischer rings[†]
  — Wilson's disease.

Carcinoid syndrome

Very rare in clinical practice. Not quite so rare in the exam.

Signs

- Hepatomegaly (knobbly, due to secondary deposits)
- Facial flushing
- Borborygmi.

The classic patient with carcinoid syndrome gives a history of flushing, diarrhoea and borborygmi. It is caused by release of 5HIAA into the systemic circulation from the secondary deposits in the liver. The primary is usually in the small bowel, appendix, duodenum or pancreas. The reason that patients with carcinoid syndrome do come up as short cases with a certain amount of regularity is that the natural history of the disease (even with secondary deposits in the liver) is often between 10 and 15 years.

Polycystic liver disease

Rare in clinical practice. Quite common in the exam.

Patients with polycystic kidney disease (p. 62) also get cysts in the liver. This can occasionally cause massive hepatomegaly, which feels knobbly/lobulated. Occasionally the hepatomegaly can be so large that the liver presses on vital organs and has to be transplanted, usually at the same time as a kidney transplant.

The main differential diagnosis of a large knobbly liver is:

- metastatic carcinoma
- carcinoid syndrome
- polycystic disease.

Patients with polycystic disease will usually also have bilateral palpable kidneys and signs of renal support such as fistulae or shunts (p. 59).

Liver transplant

The patient will have a large Mercedes-Benz type scar in the upper abdomen. There are usually no other clinical signs. There may be signs of side-effects from the immunosuppressive therapy. Such patients usually receive ciclosporin or tacrolimus, which can cause hirsutism, tremor, hypertension and renal impairment. Liver transplants have an approximately 85% 1-year survival rate and most patients who survive a year survive long term.

Indications for liver transplant include:

- acute liver failure, e.g. paracetamol overdose
- primary biliary cirrhosis
- primary sclerosing cholangitis
- autoimmune chronic active hepatitis
- hepatitis B and C
- alcoholic liver disease (must be abstinent for 6 months).

Primary biliary cirrhosis

This is an autoimmune disease with progressive inflammation and fibrosis of the intrahepatic bile ductules: 90% of cases are women; 95% have positive antimitochondrial antibodies and a raised IgM. Usually there is a gradual deterioration of liver function over 20–30 years, and transplantation is often required in the end. High-dose ursodeoxycholic acid may slow the progression of the disease.

Symptoms

- Fatigue
- Pruritus
- Jaundice (in late stages only).

Signs

- Hyperpigmentation
- Scratch marks
- Hepatosplenomegaly
- Xanthelasma and xanthoma.

Autoimmune chronic active hepatitis

This mainly affects women, usually between the ages of 15 and 30. The autoantibody is directed against the hepatocyte. Most patients are antinuclear and smooth muscle antibody-positive and have a raised IgG. The disease is very sensitive to treatment with prednisolone.

Symptoms

- Fatigue
- Nausea
- Amenorrhoea.

Signs

- Acne
- Hirsutism
- Cushingoid face
- Bruising
- Hepatosplenomegaly
- Other signs of chronic liver disease.

Crohn's disease

This is a chronic inflammatory disorder of unknown aetiology which can affect any part of the gut but has a predilection for the terminal ileum. It usually presents in patients between the ages of 20 and 40 years but can start at any age.

Symptoms

- Anorexia
- General malaise
- Abdominal pain
- Diarrhoea
- Arthralgia.

Signs

- Anaemia
- Glossitis
- Mouth ulcers
- Arthritis
- Uveitis
- Mass in the abdomen (occasionally)
- Scars from previous bowel resections
- There may be no physical signs at all.

Ulcerative colitis

This is not a common case as there are usually few physical signs.

KEY QUESTIONS

GIT

1. **What are the causes of:**
   - ascites
   - hepatomegaly
   - splenomegaly
   - hepatosplenomegaly
   - liver bruit
   - cirrhosis
   - jaundice
   - diarrhoea
   - constipation
   - anaemia
     - — hypochromic microcytic
     - — normochromic normocytic
     - — megaloblastic
   - macrocytosis (without anaemia)?
2. **What are the signs of chronic liver disease?**
3. **What is the difference clinically between splenomegaly and an enlarged left kidney?**
4. **What clinical signs might you find in a patient with chronic, active inflammatory bowel disease?**

2.5

Renal medicine

Renal medicine in the Final MB is not as frightening as it first appears. If you apply the following principles it is possible to give the examiner the impression you have spent half your life on a nephrology ward!

PRINCIPLE 1: FLUID BALANCE

If someone's kidneys do not work, that person will not pass much, if any, urine. If no urine is passed, then whatever fluid is ingested will be retained. If you or I drink 10 pints of beer one evening, we will be up all night peeing. A renal patient, however, will not form urine and so the fluid will go elsewhere, e.g.:

- lungs — pulmonary oedema
- ankles — oedema
- sacrum — oedema
- intravascular space
  - — JVP ↑
  - — BP ↑

How to assess fluid balance

	Positive balance (overloaded)	Negative balance (dry)
Skin turgor (mucous membrane)	Normal/moist	Dry
BP	↑	Postural drop
JVP	↑	↓
Lung bases	Crackles	Clear
Ankles/sacrum	Oedema	Normal

Renal patients therefore have to restrict how much fluid they take per day. Excess fluid is removed by dialysis, e.g. haemodialysis or peritoneal dialysis.

PRINCIPLE 2: DIALYSIS

If someone's kidneys do not work, renal replacement therapy (RRT) is required; this is also known as dialysis.

Haemodialysis

Blood is taken out of the body and passed through a dialysis machine before going back into the body (Fig. 2.5.1). This usually happens for 3–4 hours three times a week. Blood is taken out via a dialysis central line or a fistula (Fig. 2.5.2). A fistula is created by connecting a vein and an artery together surgically. This is then allowed to mature for several months until the vein has dilated enough for repeated cannulations.

- A fistula looks like a swollen vein, usually on the wrist or forearm. It often pulsates.
- It may have a scar over it.
- It has a machinery hum which you can hear on auscultation.

Continuous ambulatory peritoneal dialysis (CAPD)

A tube is placed surgically into the peritoneum and dialysis fluid (about 1.5 litres) passed through it. The dialysate stays in the

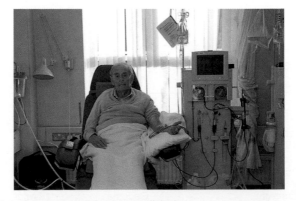

Fig. 2.5.1 A patient undergoing haemodialysis.

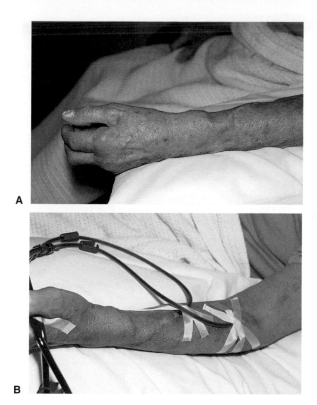

Fig. 2.5.2 A. A haemodialysis fistula. **B.** The fistula has been cannulated to allow haemodialysis.

peritoneal cavity for 4 hours, absorbing various toxins, and is then drained out so a new clean quantity of fluid can replace it. This is repeated four to five times over 24 hours. The tube is called a Tenchkoff catheter and is usually sited mid-abdomen (Fig. 2.5.3).

Causes of tubes in the abdomen

- CAPD (Tenchkoff catheter)
  — usually central
  — tube clamped, unless exchanging
  — no bag
- Ascitic drain
  — usually in flank
  — drainage bag attached
  — patient has other signs of chronic liver disease

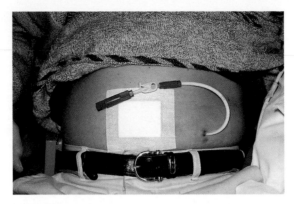

Fig. 2.5.3 A Tenchkoff catheter in situ.

- Biliary drain
  — drain usually exists in mid-axillary line over liver area
  — drainage bag attached and is usually full of bile
  — patient will often be deeply jaundiced and usually have cancer of the head of the pancreas or cholangiocarcinoma.

PRINCIPLE 3: ANAEMIA

If someone's kidneys do not work, the person is likely to be anaemic. This is because the kidney normally produces erythropoietin. Therefore, renal patients may look anaemic.

PRINCIPLE 4: URAEMIA

Patients with renal failure often have a uraemic tinge to them.

Top tip: Before finals, go down to your hospital's dialysis unit. You will notice patients' skin which has a tinge to it. Also, you can see a fistula and have a listen to it.

PRINCIPLE 5: TRANSPLANT

In an ideal world all dialysis patients would get a renal transplant. Post-transplant, such patients are likely to have a kidney-shaped lump in their left or right iliac fossa under a scar. When examining renal transplant patients, remember the following things:

- Prior to transplant they will have been on dialysis:
  — look for an old fistula
  — look for scars of old dialysis lines or Tenchkoff sites.
- Renal transplant patients will need to be on long-term immunosuppression:
  — look for evidence of steroid therapy
  — Cushingoid
  — thin skin, etc.
- Look for evidence of ciclosporin therapy:
  — gingival hypertrophy
  — hypertrichosis
  — warty skin lesions.

PRINCIPLE 6: EXAM POSSIBILITIES

Lots of people have renal failure and live active lives, thanks to renal replacement therapy. It would be easy for one of the consultants to get their dialysis patients up for the exam, as they are stable and signs are constant.

With these principles in mind, let's apply them to the likely cases you may see in finals.

Patients on haemodialysis

- Anaemic
- Uraemic tinge
- Fluid balance:
  — BP lying and standing
  — JVP
  — lung bases
  — sacrum/ankles
- Dialysis access
  — central line
  — fistulae — auscultate
  — machinery murmur.

Patients on CAPD

- Anaemic
- Uraemic
- Fluid balance — as haemodialysis
- Distended abdomen with Tenchkoff catheter in centre of abdomen
- Fluid-filled abdomen with shifting dullness.

Renal transplant patient

- Smooth kidney-shaped mass in the left or right iliac fossa
- Old abdominal scars
- Old fistula scars
- Old clavicular scars
- Cushingoid
- Signs of ciclosporin use.

Adult polycystic kidney disease (APKD)

- Enlarged ballotable abdominal masses
- Sometimes bilateral
- Sometimes associated with polycystic liver
- Check blood pressure as it is associated with hypertension
- Dipstick urine — look for haematuria
- APKD is associated with Berry aneurysms. Check scalp for craniotomy scars.

Bilateral renal enlargement: causes

- Polycystic kidney
- Bilateral hydronephrosis
- Amyloidosis.

Unilateral enlarged kidney: causes

- Hydronephrosis
- Renal cancer
- Simple renal cyst.

KEY QUESTIONS

Renal medicine

1. **Assess this patient's fluid balance.**
2. **This young man is due to go onto renal replacement therapy. Discuss with him the best choice for him.**

Haemodialysis	CAPD
Need to come into hospital three times a week	Can do it at home
Nutritional status good	Nutrition not so good
'Cleans' blood better	Less effective at 'cleaning' blood
Strict fluid balance required	Patient controls fluid balance
Need to arrange tasks around dialysis	Can do exchanges at home/work
	Peritonitis a possibility

3. **Examine this man's arms:**
   - Look for fistula
   - Feel buzz in fistula
   - Auscultate for machinery murmur.
4. **This transplant patient wants to stop taking his immunosuppressant. What advice do you have?**
   - Explore why the patient is not happy with it:
     — hassle with compliance
     — side-effects of immunosuppressant
     — problems with altered body image
     — feels well, therefore what's the point of taking tablets?
   - Explain the importance of the medicine:
     — without it, may reject kidney
     — would need dialysis again.
   - Give opportunity for questions and further discussion.
5. **Check this patient's blood pressure.**
   In a patient with a fistula, make sure you do this on the non-fistula arm!

2.6

Endocrinology

Endocrinology cases are straightforward, so long as you have prepared yourself properly for them. You will appreciate that there is no particular organ system to examine: your examination should be tailored to the patient in front of you, and may involve examining parts of several 'systems'.

TYPICAL CASES

Endocrinology

- The diabetic
- Hyperthyroidism
- Goitre
- Hypothyroidism
- Acromegaly
- Cushing's syndrome
- Addison's disease
- Hypopituitarism
- Phaeochromocytoma

The diabetic*

It would be unusual for you not to come across a diabetic patient at some stage in the exam. Diabetics are either insulin dependent (Type 1) or non-insulin dependent (Type 2).

Ask about *symptoms*:

- presenting
  — weight loss, polyuria, polydipsia, dizziness, blurred vision, etc.
- of complications
  — e.g. pins and needles (peripheral neuropathy)
  — visual problems (? new vessel formation)
  — leg ulcers (infected feet)

— vomiting
— nocturnal diarrhoea
— impotence } autonomic neuropathy
— postural hypotension
— intermittent claudication (peripheral vascular disease).

Signs

You are looking for the signs of the complications of diabetes.

Skin

- Necrobiosis lipoidica (yellow lesions on the shins, usually)
- Leg ulcers
- Infected feet/toes
- Injection sites (sometimes get fat atrophy which leaves skin hollowed out)
- Xanthelasmata (associated hyperlipidaemia)
- Granuloma annulare.

CVS

- Absent pulses in the lower limbs (peripheral vascular disease)
- Retinal changes
  - haemorrhages
  - exudates
  - new vessels
  - laser treatment
- Autonomic neuropathy (postural hypotension). This is confirmed by ECGs taken before, during and after a Valsalva manoeuvre and looking for changes in the R–R interval.

CNS

- Sensory ('glove and stocking') neuropathy
- Diabetic amyotrophy (femoral nerve damage causing wasting of quadriceps and absent knee jerk)
- Mononeuritis multiplex (multiple peripheral nerve palsies)
- Charcot's joints — painless, disorganised joint in a patient with a peripheral neuropathy.

Urogenital system. Signs of chronic renal failure (see pp. 57–63). Make sure you ask to examine the urine. You will be looking for:

1. Glucose — ? compliance with treatment; ? correct level of treatment. Ask to look at a series of urine glucoses (or BM Stix).
2. Protein — microscopic albuminuria is the first sign of diabetic renal disease, and should be carefully screened for.
3. Ketones.

You need to know about the treatment and follow-up of diabetics. Spend a couple of sessions in the diabetic clinic if you have never been.

Causes of diabetes

- Idiopathic (95%)
- Steroid therapy, thiazide diuretics
- Pancreatitis, post-pancreatectomy
- Haemochromatosis ⎫
- Cushing's syndrome ⎬ rare.
- Acromegaly, phaeochromocytoma ⎭

Hyperthyroidism

This is not a common case: most patients will be on, or have had, some form of treatment and will therefore (hopefully) be euthyroid. The diagnosis is usually given away by the typical facial appearance, with bulging eyes. However, the specific signs to look for are:

- agitation, sweating
- tremor (exaggerated physiological tremor)
- resting tachycardia
- atrial fibrillation
- exophthalmos
- lid lag/lid retraction
- goitre
- bruit over the thyroid
- pretibial myxoedema ⎫
- proximal myopathy ⎬ rare.

Goitre

You may be asked to 'examine this patient's goitre'. Follow the simple scheme of:

1. look
2. feel

3. percuss (retrosternal goitre)
4. listen.

Look at the contours of the patient's neck from the front and the side. If it is a goitre there will be a swelling between the thyroid cartilage and the manubrium sterni. It may be mainly unilateral, particularly if there is a single nodule in the thyroid.

Now go behind the patient to palpate the thyroid with the flat of both hands (best done with the patient sitting in a chair). Ask the patient to have a sip from a glass of water and hold the water in the mouth. When you are ready, ask the patient to swallow while palpating the thyroid. If the swelling goes up on swallowing, the diagnosis is that of a goitre.

Now assess the characteristics of the goitre:

- smooth
  — Graves' disease
  — simple goitre (iodine-deficient)
  — multiple cysts
  — multinodular goitre
- single nodule
  — carcinoma of the thyroid
  — benign adenoma
  — single simple cyst
- tender
  — thyroiditis.

If you feel a single nodule, feel for local lymph nodes and attachment to local structures in the neck. These are features of a malignant thyroid nodule. Remember to listen for a bruit over the thyroid (ask the patient to hold the breath). This is sometimes heard in Graves' disease with a very vascular thyroid. You must now look for signs of hyper- or hypothyroidism.

Hypothyroidism

Again this is not a common examination case, for reasons given above.

Causes

- Idiopathic atrophy
- Post-^{131}I therapy

- Post-thyroidectomy
- Post-Hashimoto's thyroiditis.

Signs

- Psychomotor retardation
- Dry scaly skin
- 'Peaches and cream' complexion
- Dry brittle hair, hair loss
- Loss of outer third of eyebrow (unreliable sign)
- Goitre
- Hoarse voice
- Weight gain
- Sinus bradycardia
- Carpal tunnel syndrome
- Slow-relaxing reflexes
- Cardiomyopathy
- Dementia
- Peripheral neuropathy   } rare.
- Cerebellar degeneration

Acromegaly

This is caused by a growth hormone-secreting adenoma in the pituitary gland. Even after treatment with bromocriptine or hypophysectomy (or both) the patient will still have residual signs of the disease. So, although acromegaly is a rare condition in everyday clinical practice, it is relatively common in the examination setting.

Signs

- Prominent jaw, nose, orbital ridges
- Large hands
- Large feet
- Typical facies
- Large, burly stature.

Remember to examine the visual fields for bitemporal hemianopia, which is caused by a local pressure effect of the tumour on the optic chiasm.

Complications of acromegaly

- Hypertension
- Proximal myopathy
- Carpal tunnel syndrome
- Osteoarthrosis (particularly of lower limbs)
- Cardiomyopathy (this is not infrequently the cause of death in the patient's 50s or 60s).

Associated conditions

- Diabetes
- Hypopituitarism
- Hypercalcaemia.

Cushing's syndrome

This syndrome is due to excess circulating corticosteroids.

Causes

- Iatrogenic* — Patients with conditions such as asthma or systemic lupus erythematosus are not infrequently treated with oral steroids and may exhibit some of the signs of Cushing's syndrome.
- Cushing's disease — ACTH-secreting pituitary adenoma[†].
- Adrenal cortical adenoma.
- Ectopic ACTH from bronchial carcinoma[†].

The commonest cause, by far, is the iatrogenic variety.

Signs

- Moon face
- Fragile skin
- Easy bruising
- Buffalo hump
- Striae (abdominal wall)
- Hirsutism
- Muscular wasting
- Proximal myopathy.

Patients with Cushing's syndrome are more likely to develop diabetes, hypertension, recurrent infections and bone fractures (osteoporotic).

Note. Nelson's syndrome occurs after adrenalectomy for Cushing's disease. The main features are of pigmentation associated with the increase in circulating ACTH which follows such an operation.

Addison's disease[t]

In this condition there are insufficient circulating corticosteroids due to failure of the adrenal cortex. You will not see an untreated case in the exam. The patient may have been on treatment for many years and usually will have no clinical signs.

Causes

- Idiopathic* — autoimmune and associated with diabetes and thyroid disease
- Metastatic deposits in the adrenal cortex from a primary in the lung or breast
- Tuberculosis[t] — calcified adrenals on plain abdominal X-ray.

Symptoms

- Weight loss
- Lassitude
- Postural hypotension
- Visual disturbance
- Vomiting.

Signs

- Pigmentation
  - hand (palmar creases)
  - knee
  - buccal
  - generalised
- Postural hypotension
- Fluid depletion.

The urea and electrolytes show hyponatraemia and hyperkalaemia.

Hypopituitarism[†]

Rare case.

Phaeochromocytoma[†]

Very rare exam case.

KEY QUESTIONS

Endocrinology

1. What are the causes of:
   - diabetes
   - goitre
   - Cushing's syndrome
   - Addison's disease?
2. What clinical features suggest a malignant goitre?
3. Describe the more unusual ways in which the following diseases may present:
   - diabetes
   - thyrotoxicosis
   - hypothyroidism
   - Addison's disease
   - Cushing's disease.
4. What abnormalities are found in the serum glucose and urea and electrolytes in:
   - Addison's disease
   - Cushing's disease?
5. What are the clinical features of panhypopituitarism?

Neurology

Neurological cases are regarded with some trepidation by many candidates. There are several reasons for this. Neurological disease can result in many signs, some of which carry rather long and unpronounceable names. A good neurological examination is an art form: when performed by an expert it can be a pleasure to watch. This is rarely the case in the examination room.

Candidates are sometimes wrong-footed by the question 'where is the lesion?'. Unfortunately, to give a meaningful answer you need to understand basic neuroanatomy. Before you start this chapter, therefore, we recommend you acquaint yourself with the following information from a standard anatomy textbook:

- sensory pathways
- motor pathways
- sensory dermatomes
- root values of:
  — peripheral nerves
  — muscle groups
  — reflex arcs
- gross anatomy of the brain, including brain stem, cranial nerves and their nuclei.

The most important thing to remember about a neurological examination is that it is *comparative*. In other words you test one sign on one side and then test on the other side and compare the difference. Do not forget to do this at all times: the examiners will be looking closely for it.

In the examination room you will rarely, if ever, be asked to do a full neurological examination in the clinical skills OSCEs — this would take far too long. Instead, the examiner will ask you to examine part of the nervous system (e.g. arms, legs, cranial nerves, cerebellum, etc.).

You must be practised at doing such bits of a full neurological examination. It is for this reason that this chapter has been divided into the sections of 'regional neurology' as set out below:

Table 2.7.1 Differences between UMN and LMN lesions

	UMN	LMN
Observation	—	Wasting, fasciculation
Tone	Spasticity	Hypotonicity
Power	Weakness	Weakness
Reflexes	Hyperreflexia	Hyporeflexia
	Extensor plantars	
	Clonus	

- The head
  - — eyes
  - — cranial nerves
  - — speech
  - — higher functions
- Upper limb
- Lower limb
- Abnormal gait and movements
- Diffuse disease.

Many neurological problems will extend beyond the region you have been asked to examine. You must appreciate this and be seen to appreciate it by the examiners. For example, if you find ataxic nystagmus when asked to examine the eyes, you must be seen to look for other signs of multiple sclerosis.

Before you start the rest of the chapter it is important to appreciate the difference between upper motor neurone (UMN) and lower motor neurone (LMN) lesions. This is a frequently asked question (see Table 2.7.1).

Try to look stylish when you swing the patella hammer.

THE HEAD

EYES

Examination of the eyes causes mortal fear in some candidates. Actually this is unnecessary: eye cases are usually rather simple. You need to have a good scheme for examination, a grasp of the essentials of using an ophthalmoscope and a knowledge of the cases which you are likely to meet.

Scheme for the examination of the eyes

Observation

Look at the patient's eyes at rest. The diagnosis may be obvious, e.g. exophthalmos (thyrotoxicosis), Horner's syndrome, etc. (see Fig. 2.7.1). Also look for xanthelasmata, senile arcus, etc.

Feel

Feel for increased tone in the eyes (palpation). This is a very inaccurate way of assessing intraocular pressure, which is normally measured by a very sensitive machine. Intraocular pressure is raised in conditions such as glaucoma.

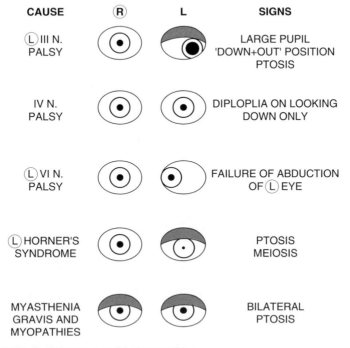

CAUSE	Ⓡ	L	SIGNS
Ⓛ III N. PALSY			LARGE PUPIL 'DOWN+OUT' POSITION PTOSIS
IV N. PALSY			DIPLOPLIA ON LOOKING DOWN ONLY
Ⓛ VI N. PALSY			FAILURE OF ABDUCTION OF Ⓛ EYE
Ⓛ HORNER'S SYNDROME			PTOSIS MEIOSIS
MYASTHENIA GRAVIS AND MYOPATHIES			BILATERAL PTOSIS

Fig. 2.7.1 Pupillary and eyelid abnormalities.

Visual acuity

Test this by asking the patient to read some small print (with glasses if worn), e.g. from a newspaper. A more formal assessment can be made with standard Snellen charts.

Visual fields

Sit on the edge of the patient's bed. Equilibrate the patient's visual fields with your own by making sure your heads are at the same level, 1 metre apart. Ask the patient to cover one eye. Now cover your own eye (the opposite one to the one the patient has just covered). Test the patient's visual field (against your own) by slowly bringing a finger or white hat-pin from outside your field of vision (while the patient looks into your uncovered eye). Bring the hat-pin in at 2, 4, 8 and 10 o'clock, as this will pick up quadrantic field defects better. Now, using a red hat-pin, assess the blind spot (against your own) and look for scotomata (see common field defects, Fig. 2.7.2).

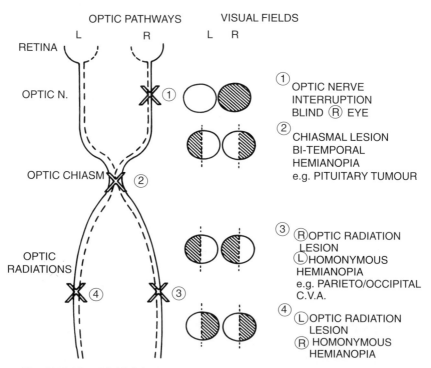

Fig. 2.7.2 Visual field defects.

Fundoscopy

It is essential to be familiar with the ophthalmoscope you use during the examination. The only way to ensure that this happens is by taking your own or one you have borrowed. The patient should be in a darkened room with dilated pupils (ask for mydriatic drops if necessary). Set the machine with a plain lens and normal filters. Shine it onto your hand to check it is working. Now elicit the red reflex in both the patient's eyes. This is done by shining the light through the pupil from about 0.5 m. Light hits the retina and is reflected back as a red glow as you look through the lens of the ophthalmoscope. Anything which causes an interruption to this pathway of light will cause an absent red reflex, e.g.:

- cataract
- prosthetic eye
- haemorrhage into anterior chamber
- vitreous haemorrhage.

Now examine the eye itself. Start off by asking the patient to look at a spot in the distance, ignoring the light of the ophthalmoscope. Approach the patient's eye from a slightly lateral direction. This approach has two advantages:

1. It enables the patient to concentrate on the spot in the distance, with minimal disturbance to the field of vision.
2. The optic disc should pop straight into view.

Focus on the optic disc by altering the lens strength to get a sharp image. For short-sighted patients you will need a negative lens and for long-sighted patients you will need a positive lens. Once you have found the disc your problems should be over. Examine it carefully and assess:

- colour
- margin
- contour.

If you cannot find the disc, follow the vessels until it comes into view. Now look at all areas of the retina and in particular:

- vessels
  - tortuosity
  - silver wiring
  - a-v nipping
  - new vessel formation
  - haemorrhages

- retinal surface
  — haemorrhages
  — exudates
  — evidence of laser therapy.

Now slowly 'rack back' by increasing the lens strength of the oph-thalmoscope. Check the posterior chamber, lens (for cataracts) and anterior chamber. With practice, fundoscopy will become easier. Examine as many normal fundi as possible. Remember that the retinae of Blacks and Asians look much darker than those of Caucasians.

Move

You will be essentially testing cranial nerves III, IV and VI and the intraocular muscles which they supply. Stand to the left of the patient. Rest your left hand on the patient's forehead (to help keep it still). Now, asking the patient to follow the index finger of your right hand, test all directions of movement. Ask the patient to say 'yes' if he or she sees double. Try to find out in which direction of gaze the double vision is worst. Look for:

- failure of gaze (and direction)
- nystagmus
- dysconjugate gaze.

Note. Make sure you do not confuse physiological and patho-logical nystagmus. To avoid this mistake remember the following two tips:

- Do not draw the patient's gaze too far laterally.
- Do not place the finger too close to the patient's eyes (0.5 m is usually ideal).

TYPICAL CASES

Neurology — eyes

- Fundoscopy
- Ptosis
- Horner's syndrome
- Large pupil
- Small pupil
- Nystagmus

Fundoscopy

Normal appearance of fundus

It would be a bit naughty of the examiner to give you a normal fundus (see Fig. 2.7.3). However, until you know what is or isn't normal, fundoscopy will prove difficult.

Optic atrophy

If the disc looks surprisingly white, distinct and much easier to find than normal, it is probably optic atrophy (Fig. 2.7.4). It is absolutely essential to compare it with the disc on the other side.

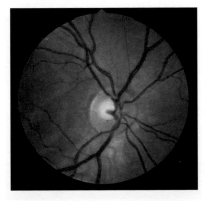

Fig. 2.7.3 Normal fundus.

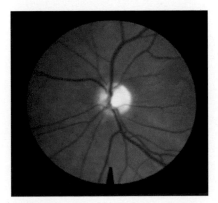

Fig. 2.7.4 Optic atrophy.

Causes

- Multiple sclerosis
- Post-traumatic
- Retro-orbital tumour
- Diabetes
- Retinal artery thrombosis.

Proliferative diabetic retinopathy

The reason new vessels occur in the diabetic fundus is due to retinal ischaemia. It is important to recognise NVD (Fig. 2.7.5), as, untreated, such patients rapidly go blind. Figure 2.7.6 shows the condition with new vessels elsewhere (NVE).

Other signs commonly seen in the diabetic eye include:

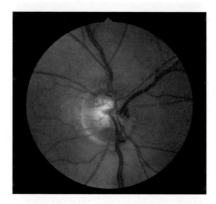

Fig. 2.7.5 Proliferative diabetic retinopathy with new vessels on disc (NVD).

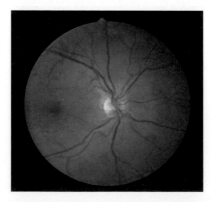

Fig. 2.7.6 Proliferative diabetic retinopathy with new vessels elsewhere (NVE).

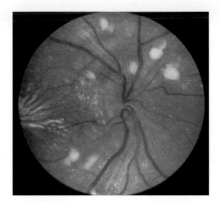

Fig. 2.7.7 Severe hypertensive retinopathy with papilloedema.

- haemorrhages
- exudates
- cataracts.

Severe hypertensive retinopathy with papilloedema

Hypertensive retinopathy is classified as severe if papilloedema is present. Severe hypertensive retinopathy is usually seen in young or middle-aged patients with accelerated hypertension, often of renal origin (e.g. glomerulonephritis). Figure 2.7.7 shows some of the other changes seen in the fundus in hypertensives, including arteriolar narrowing, hard and soft exudates.

Causes (of papilloedema)

- Accelerated hypertension
- Benign intracranial hypertension
- Raised intracranial pressure (any cause).

Top tip: if you find the disc difficult or impossible to find, papilloedema is probably present.

Retinitis pigmentosa

Figure 2.7.8 shows the classical 'bone spicule' appearance around the periphery of the retina. The purple spot at the fovea is artefactual (caused by the light reflex when the photograph was taken).

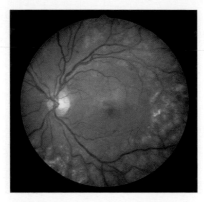

Fig. 2.7.8 Retinitis pigmentosa.

Fig. 2.7.9 Fundoscopic appearance of a glass eye.

Retinitis pigmentosa is a genetic disorder and may be autosomal dominant, autosomal recessive or X-linked. As the peripheral part of the retina is affected first, patients may present with night blindness and tunnel vision. Central vision acuity is relatively spared in the early stages of the disease. Most patients are registered blind by their 30s, although this is variable and depends to some extent on the genetic type.

Glass eye

Some nasty examiners will ask you to perform fundoscopy on a prosthetic eye (Fig. 2.7.9). If you remember to do the red reflex first you will stay one step ahead.

Ptosis (drooping of the eyelid)

Causes

- Third nerve palsy (large pupil)
- Part of Horner's syndrome (small pupil)
- Myopathies (usually bilateral ptosis)
  — myaesthenia gravis
  — myotonia congenita
  — other congenital myopathies, e.g. facio/scapulohumeral
  — idiopathic.

Note. Bilateral ptosis, particularly if mild, can be difficult to spot.

Horner's syndrome

This is rare in practice, but common in exams. There is a classical combination of signs, which is:

- ptosis
- enophthalmos
- meiosis (small pupil)
- ipsilateral loss of sweating (face).

It is caused by interruption of the sympathetic supply to levator palpebrae superioris and dilator pupillae. This can be caused by lesions in the brain stem, stellate ganglion or root of neck.

Causes

- Carcinoma of bronchus (Pancoast's tumour)
- Syringomyelia (UMN signs in legs, LMN signs in arms)
- Syringobulbia (bulbar palsy)
- Sympathectomy
- Tumour at root of neck, cervical cord.

Large pupil

Causes

- Mydriatic drops*
- Holmes–Adie pupil* (dilated pupil, which responds very slowly to light, plus absent ankle jerks in young females)
- Third nerve palsy
- Surgical (irregular pupil) iridectomy, cataract removal.

Small pupil

Causes

- Old age*
- Horner's syndrome
- Pilocarpine (treatment for glaucoma)
- Argyll Robertson pupil[†] (irregular pupil) with absent light reflex found in syphilis.

Nystagmus

Describe it in terms of the fast phase of movement.

Horizontal nystagmus — causes

- Vestibular causes (associated with deafness and vertigo)
  — Ménière's disease
  — middle ear surgery
  — multiple sclerosis
  — syringobulbia
  — viral labyrinthitis
- Cerebellar causes (look for other cerebellar signs)
  — tumour, primary or secondary
  — degenerative disease
  — multiple sclerosis
  — cerebrovascular disease.

THE CRANIAL NERVES

The examiners may ask you to examine the whole lot, but more often they will select a single cranial nerve for you to examine. This is most often the VIIth cranial nerve (see Table 2.7.2).

Scheme for examining the cranial nerves

II

- Acuity
- Visual fields   see (74–84)
- Fundoscopy

III, IV, VI (see p. 75)

VII*

Test the facial muscles:

- Orbicularis oculi ('screw your eyes up tight and don't let me open them')
- Orbicularis oris ('smile, keep your lips together and don't let me open them')
- Frontalis muscle ('raise your eyebrows').

This last test distinguishes an upper motor neurone (UMN) VIIth lesion from a lower motor neurone (LMN) VIIth lesion. In the latter there is total 'face drop', including frontalis (forehead). In a UMN VIIth nerve lesion the forehead is spared, because of bilateral cortical representation of the frontalis muscle. This is a very commonly asked question.

Summary. UMN VII, forehead spared; LMN VII, total face drop.

Examination of the other cranial nerves is summarised in Table 2.7.2.

SPEECH

Dysarthria

This is a difficulty in the physical articulation of the spoken word caused by a failure of the elements of the speech 'end organ' (i.e. a local cause). There are degrees of dysarthria, and mild dysarthria can be made more pronounced by one of the standard tongue-twisters: 'West Register Street'; 'baby hippopotamus'.

Causes

- Ill-fitting dentures*
- Cranial nerve palsy VII, IX, X, XII
- Bulbar palsy
- Pseudobulbar palsy ('hot potato' speech)
- Cerebellar disease ('staccato' speech).

Bulbar palsy is caused by bilateral LMN lesions of cranial nerves IX, X, XII. Patients often complain of nasal regurgitation. Signs include fasciculating tongue and loss of gag reflex. It is rare and usually caused by motor neurone disease.

Table 2.7.2 Cranial nerve palsies

Cranial nerve	Sign	Causes
I[†]	Smell (bottles)	Frontal lobe tumour
		Fractured skull
II	Visual fields	MS
	• scotomata	Retro-orbital tumour
	• field loss (Fig. 2.7.2)	Alcohol
	Fundoscopy	Tobacco
	• papillitis	Macular degeneration
	• optic atrophy	
	Pupillar reflexes	
	• visual acuity	
III	Ptosis, large pupil, eye deviation (down and out)	Cavernous sinus thrombosis
IV[†]	Diplopia on downward gaze	Raised intracranial pressure
VI	Failure of lateral gaze (Fig. 2.7.1)	
V[†] motor	Jaw deviates to side of lesion	
sensory	Anaesthetic area (depends on branch affected) reduced corneal reflex (V[1])	Cerebellopontine angle tumour
VII*	Ipsilateral face drop	Idiopathic (Bell's palsy)
	Bell's sign (LMN only)	Middle ear
		• tumour
		• infection
		Post-surgical
		Sarcoid (sometimes bilateral)
VIII[†]	Weber and Rinne tests (see notes)	Wax
		Otitis media } Conductive
		Otosclerosis } deafness
		Trauma
		Infection } Perceptive
		VIII nerve } deafness
		tumour } (sensorineural)
		Streptomycin

Table 2.7.2 (*continued*)

IX ⎫	Uvula deviates away from affected side	*Unilateral lesion*
X ⎬		Tumour or deposits around jugular foramen
XI	Reduced bulk of trapezius	
	Reduced power on shrugging shoulders and sternocleidomastoid	
XII	Ipsilateral wasting of tongue	*Bilateral lesions*
	Deviation of tongue to affected side	Syringobulbia
	Tongue fasciculation	Motor neurone disease (MND)

Notes to Table 2.7.2

1. When examining the VIIth nerve: if you think it is an LMN lesion, always look behind the ipsilateral ear and over the ipsilateral parotid for scars (mastoid and parotid surgery, respectively). These are common causes of this problem, and will make your examination look classy.
2. Look for Bell's sign (LMN VIIth). On attempted eye closure, the ipsilateral eye deviates upwards.
3. The following can cause any cranial nerve lesion:
   - diabetes
   - multiple sclerosis (MS)
   - sarcoid
   - nerve tumour
   - post-meningitis.
4. *Rinne's test*. Hold a tuning fork on the mastoid process until it is no longer audible. Now hold it by the external auditory canal: in the normal ear it should now be audible (air conduction [AC] > bone conduction [BC]). In perceptive deafness (VIIIth nerve problem) this situation persists. In conductive deafness BC > AC because air-conducted sound depends on intact auditory ossicles for its transmission.
5. *Weber's test*. Place a tuning fork on the vertex of the skull. In normal people it is heard equally well in both ears. In sensory deafness the tuning fork will not be heard in the affected ear. In conductive deafness, the noise will be heard equally well in both ears. This is because the auditory ossicles are bypassed by direct bone conduction.

Pseudobulbar palsy is caused by bilateral UMN lesions (e.g. bilateral CVAs). It is more common than a true bulbar palsy. Patients complain of nasal regurgitation and relatives may say that the patient cries inappropriately (labile emotions). They have a characteristic speech which is high-pitched but rather nasal ('hot potato' or 'Donald Duck' speech). In addition they have a positive jaw jerk and may have bilateral UMN signs in the limbs.

Dysphasia

There are two types of dysphasia, expressive (or nominal) and receptive.

In *expressive dysphasia*, which is due to a lesion in Broca's motor speech area (frontoparietal), there is a failure of speech content or expression. This results in the patient being unable to name familiar objects such as a pen, jacket, etc., while knowing what they are. Its usual cause is a CVA in the dominant hemisphere.

Receptive dysphasia is due to failure of integration of hearing and speech. This results in the patient being unable to understand the spoken word. It is usually caused by a CVA or other lesion in Wernicke's area of the dominant hemisphere (temporoparietal).

Aphasia is the inability to speak at all.

Patients with both expressive and receptive dysphasia will be unable to name familiar objects. The way to quickly distinguish the two types of dysphasia is as follows:

Q. 'Can you tell me what this is?' (show the patient a pen).
   Neither will give a meaningful reply.
Q. 'Is it a watch?'
   Receptive dysphasic: no meaningful reply.
   Expressive dysphasic: 'No!'
Q. 'Is it a key?'
   Receptive dysphasic: no meaningful reply.
   Expressive dysphasic: 'No!'
Q. 'Is it a pen?'
   Receptive dysphasic: no meaningful reply.
   Expressive dysphasic: 'Yes!'

HIGHER FUNCTIONS

General cerebral function

Patients with a generalised systemic disease or generalised disease of cerebral substance often have intellectual impairment. You ought to have a list of questions at your fingertips to demonstrate such problems:

— name	— dates of Second World War
— age	— time
— address	— recent newsworthy events
— date of birth	— day of week
— name of monarch	— date
— name of prime minister	— place of interview?

Additional tests such as ability to remember three objects, ability to serially subtract 7 from 100 and ability to remember a six figure number can also be valuable.

Frontal lobe function[†]

Patients with frontal lobe problems tend to be disinhibited. They may wander. They are frequently incontinent. Valuable information is gained from relatives/neighbours.

Parietal lobe function[†]

On a superficial examination there may be no abnormalities, unless specifically looked for:

- sensory inattention (non-dominant hemisphere)
- apraxia (loss of fine movements associated with a complicated task, e.g. dressing, retrieving a match from a closed matchbox)
- astereognosis (inability to recognise object placed in hand with eyes closed)
- dyslexia (reading difficulties)
- dysgraphia (writing difficulties)
- dyscalculia (mathematical difficulties)
- left/right disorientation
- finger agnosia (inability to recognise objects by touch).

THE UPPER LIMB

Scheme for the examination of the upper limb

Observation

- Wasting ⎫
- Fasciculation ⎬ LMN lesions
- Posture, e.g. 'waiter's tip', 'claw hand'
- Scars, e.g. ulnar nerve transposition.

Tone

- Increased (UMN)
- Decreased (LMN)
- Cogwheel (extrapyramidal).

Power

Root values	Movement
C3, 4	Shoulder abduction
C5, 6	Shoulder adduction
	Elbow flexion
C7	Elbow ⎫
	Wrist ⎬ Extension
	Finger ⎭
C8, T1	Small muscles of hand

Peripheral nerve motor supply

- Ulnar: all small muscles of hand with the exception of 'LOAF' (median nerve) muscles
- Median
  - **L**ateral two lumbricals (flexion of M/P joints)
  - **O**pponens pollicis
  - **A**bductor pollicis
  - **F**lexor pollicis brevis
- Radial: wrist and finger extensors.

Sensation

Test:

- pain (pinprick)
- light touch (cotton wool)
- joint position sense
- vibration (tuning fork).

Temperature sensation is usually irrelevant in the exam.

You must map out the area of sensory loss and try to deduce whether it is a root or peripheral nerve problem. Remember to compare the sides (see Figs 2.7.10 and 2.7.11 for sensory supply of upper limb).

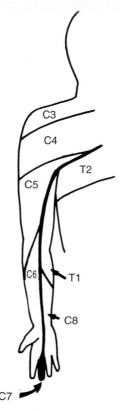

Fig. 2.7.10 Sensory dermatomes: upper limbs. C7 is the key to working it out; this supplies middle finger of hand. Note the C4/T2 interface on the upper chest wall.

Reflexes

Reflex	Root
Biceps	C5, 6
Supinator	C6
Triceps	C7, 8

Cerebellar signs

- Past pointing
- Intention tremor
- Dysdiadochokinesis.

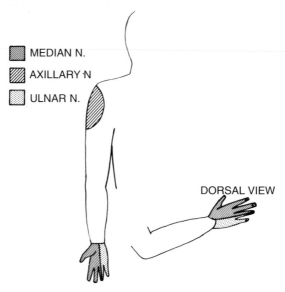

Fig. 2.7.11 Distribution of sensory loss in peripheral nerve lesions: upper limbs. *Note*. Radial nerve palsies often result in no demonstrable sensory loss (overlapping nerve supply). Patients sometimes complain of paraesthesiae over dorsum of thumb.

Involuntary movements

- Tremor
- Athetosis
- Chorea
- Ballismus.

TYPICAL CASES

Neurology — the upper limb

- The wasted hand
- Ulnar nerve palsy
- Median nerve palsy
- Radial nerve palsy
- Nerve to serratus anterior
- C5, C6 root
- T1 root (Klumpke's palsy)
- UMN signs

- LMN signs
- Sensory problems
- Proximal myopathy
- Parkinson's syndrome
- Cerebellar signs

The wasted hand*

Very common case. There are many causes of wasting of the small muscles of the hand:
- non-neurological
  - old age*
  - rheumatoid arthritis*
- neurological
  - cervical rib
  - T1 root lesion
  - ulnar nerve palsy
  - syringomyelia ⎫ Often
  - motor neurone disease ⎭ bilateral signs.

Try to ascertain the cause. Remember that MND and syringomyelia may have UMN signs in the legs. Look for scars around the elbow (ulnar nerve palsy). It can be difficult to sort out whether it is a T1 root lesion or an ulnar palsy. Table 2.7.3 will help.

Ulnar nerve palsy

Usually at the elbow, often traumatic (Table 2.7.3).

Median nerve palsy*

Very common. It will usually be due to carpal tunnel syndrome.

Table 2.7.3 Ulnar nerve and T1 root palsies		
	Power	*Sensory loss*
T1 root	Reduced in all small muscles of hand	Often little
Ulnar nerve	LOAF not affected (median nerve supply)	Inner aspect of medial $1\frac{1}{2}$ fingers and inner aspect of forearm

Signs

- Reduced power in LOAF
- Sensory loss lateral $3\frac{1}{2}$ fingers
- Tinel's sign (tapping over median nerve at the wrist causes paraesthesiae).

Causes of carpal tunnel syndrome

- Myxoedema
- Acromegaly
- Rheumatoid arthritis
- Pregnancy
- Trauma.

It is most common in middle-aged women with none of the above.

Radial nerve palsy

Wrist drop due to radial nerve palsy (usually) as it passes through the spiral groove. Finger extension and elbow extension are also reduced. It is common in alcoholics and for this reason is also known as 'Saturday night palsy'. After a Saturday night binge, the patient falls sound asleep in the armchair while watching TV, the arms having flopped over the edge of the chair. In this position the radial nerve (in the spiral groove) is exposed to trauma from the arm of the chair. Next morning, on awakening, the arm is fairly useless (try to use your own fingers with your wrist fully flexed!), but usually recovers spontaneously.

Nerve to serratus anterior (C5, 6, 7)[†]

Causes 'winging of the scapula'.

C5, C6 root (Erb–Duchenne palsy)

Causes

- Birth trauma
- Falling from a motorbike onto the tip of the shoulder.

Signs

- Posture — 'waiter tip sign' (the arm is held internally rotated with flexion of the metacarpophalangeal joints)

- Reduced sensation on outer aspect of the arm
- Absent biceps and supinator jerks
- C5, 6 motor loss (see earlier).

T1 root (Klumpke's palsy)

Causes

- Birth trauma
- Trauma
- Cervical rib
- Pancoast's tumour.

Signs

- Wasted hand (clawed)
- Sensory loss on inner aspect of upper arm.

UMN signs

- Unilateral
  — e.g. CVA
  — cerebral tumour
- Bilateral
  — e.g. bilateral CVAs
  — MS
  — high cord lesion
  — syringobulbia
  — motor neurone disease (often LMN signs predominate in upper limbs).

LMN signs

- Unilateral* (see first seven cases, pp. 93–95)
- Bilateral
  — syringomyelia
  — MND
  — bilateral cervical ribs.

Sensory problems†

Sensory signs are usually found in conjunction with motor signs, as already outlined. It is extremely rare to get a peripheral sensory neuropathy which solely affects the hands: symptoms in the lower limbs usually predominate.

Proximal myopathy[†]

Weakness of proximal muscles. Patients find difficulty in raising their arms (e.g. combing the hair).

Causes

- Polymyositis
- Dermatomyositis — heliotrope rash under eyes/erythematous rash over hands (50% have an underlying carcinoma)
- Cushing's syndrome
- Thyrotoxicosis
- Carcinoma
- Diabetes
- Hereditary.

Don't forget to check the power in the proximal muscles of the legs as these are often affected (inability to stand from the sitting position with the arms folded across the chest).

Parkinson's syndrome (see pp. 102–103)

Cerebellar signs (see pp. 103–104)

THE LOWER LIMB

Scheme for examination of the lower limb

Use the same routine as that for the upper limb.

Inspection

- Wasting
- Scars
- Foot drop, etc.

Tone

Power

Root	Muscle group
L1, 2	Hip flexion
L3, 4	Knee extension
L5, S1	Knee flexion
L4, L5	Ankle dorsiflexion
S1	Ankle plantarflexion

Reflexes

- Knee — L3, 4
- Ankle — L5, S1.
  Knee and ankle clonus are found in upper motor neurone lesions.

Sensory assessment (see Fig. 2.7.12)

Remember that sensory dermatomes in the lower limb are rather less clearcut than in the upper limbs.

Coordination

- Heel/shin test.

Romberg's test

Ask the patient to close the eyes while standing. Romberg's test is positive if the patient now falls over. It is a test of dorsal column function.

Gait (see pp. 101–104)

TYPICAL CASES

Neurology — the lower limb

- Sensory neuropathy
- Foot drop

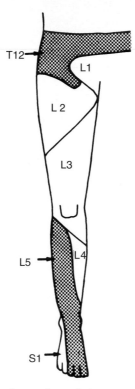

Fig. 2.7.12 Sensory dermatomes: lower limbs.

- Root lesions
- Unilateral UMN signs
- Bilateral UMN signs
- Hereditary sensory motor neuropathies

Sensory neuropathy*

Common case. Symmetrical sensation loss. All modalities affected. 'Glove and stocking' distribution, but lower limbs affected first and more severely.

Causes

- Alcohol*
- Diabetes*

- Carcinomatosis*
- Drugs (e.g. nitrofurantoin)
- Vitamin deficiency (especially the B group).

Rare causes: Guillain–Barré syndrome, amyloid, sarcoid, uraemia, myeloma, porphyria, leprosy.
   Remember to look for the consequences of neuropathy, e.g.:

- painless ulcers
- Charcot's joints (ankle, knee).

Foot drop

Lateral peroneal nerve palsy. It is often caused by trauma to the head of the fibula (bumper-bar injury) but can be found spontaneously in diabetics.

Signs

- Foot drop
- High stepping gait on affected side
- Sensory examination
- Reflexes } normal.

Other causes of foot drop

- Mononeuritis multiplex
- Peripheral neuropathy
- Motor neurone disease
- Peroneal muscular atrophy (Charcot–Marie–Tooth syndrome).

Root lesions[†]

L5

- Weakness of extensors of the great toe
- Reduced/absent ankle jerk
- Reduced sensation over L5 dermatome.

S1

- Reduced power
  — plantarflexion
  — foot eversion

- Absent ankle jerk
- Reduced sensation over outer aspect of foot.

L2–4

These root lesions are very rare. They are caused by:
- prolapsed intervertebral disc*
- metastases
- meningioma.

Unilateral UMN signs*

Found in common-or-garden cerebrovascular accidents.

Bilateral UMN signs (spastic paraparesis)

Rare in practice, common in examinations.

Signs

- Bilateral
  — hypertonia
  — hyperreflexia
  — plantar extensors
  — ankle/knee clonus
  — weakness
  — sensory loss.

You *must* look for a 'sensory level' (use a pin on abdominal and thoracic walls). This will tell you the level of the lesion in the spinal cord.

Causes

- Trauma (usually RTA)
- Vertebral collapse
  — metastatic cancer
  — osteoporosis
- Tumours
  — *extradural*
    — meningioma

— angioma
— neurofibroma
— metastases
— *intrinsic*, e.g. glioma
- Spinal artery embolism
- Multiple sclerosis
- Motor neurone disease
- Syringomyelia/bulbia.

Hereditary sensory motor neuropathies[†]

Peroneal muscular atrophy. Types I and II used to be known as 'Charcot–Marie–Tooth' disease.

Rare case. Autosomal dominant condition causing wasting of peroneal muscles in early adult life. Eventually all the lower leg muscles waste, causing the 'inverted champagne bottle' appearance.

Signs

- Wasting
- Foot drop
- Impaired vibration sense and general sensory loss
- Signs in the upper limbs (very rare).

ABNORMAL GAIT AND MOVEMENTS

ABNORMAL GAIT

Cerebrovascular accident (CVA)*

There is a rigid leg and partially plantarflexed foot. The patient drags the leg through a semicircle.

Spastic paraplegia

The patient drags both spastic legs. He usually swings the upper torso to help him move. This has been described as a 'wading through mud gait'.

Dorsal column loss

The patient looks at the ground. He has a wide-based gait with high foot lift. The patient will fall if the eyes are closed (Romberg's sign). The patient may also have loss of joint position and vibration sense.

Causes

- Diabetes
- Friedreich's ataxia
- Subacute combined degeneration of the cord } rare.
- Tabes dorsalis

Foot drop gait

High stepping gait. Feet slap the ground.

Causes

- Lateral peroneal nerve palsy
- Poliomyelitis
- Charcot–Marie–Tooth disease
- Motor neurone disease.

Proximal myopathy

Waddling gait (looks like a duck). The upper torso swings to aid forward propulsion of the limbs. The patient will have difficulty getting out of a chair (see p. 96).

Parkinson's disease*

Shuffling gait. Small steps. The patient is stooped and rigid, and finds turning difficult. The arms do not swing. Festination (sudden increase in speed of walking). On/off phenomenon (patient suddenly 'freezes' during a movement — a most distressing symptom). Patients with Parkinson's disease find initiating movements difficult. Remember to assess how the patient's illness affects daily life, e.g. dressing (buttons may be impossible), eating, etc.

Other signs

- Tremor
  - 6 Hz
  - pill rolling
  - better during voluntary action
- Bradykinesia
  - facial immobility
- Rigidity (cogwheel).

Causes

- Idiopathic.
- Drugs, e.g. major tranquillisers.
- Drug abuse, e.g. MTPT.
- Vascular (multiple CVAs to the basal ganglia). This variety is usually unresponsive to therapy.
- Post-viral (encephalitis lethargica occurred in the early 1920s — all of these patients are now dead).
- Repeated trauma, e.g. boxers.

Cerebellar disease

Veering gait. Patients fall to side of the lesion (this is accentuated by asking the patient to walk along an imaginary white line on the floor).

Other signs (all ipsilateral)

- Dysarthria
- Nystagmus (fast phase to side of lesion)
- Intention tremor (this is an oscillating tremor which is worse on movement)
- Past pointing (finger–nose test)
- Dysdiadochokinesis
- Poor heel/shin test
- Cerebellar drift (when the patient holds the hands outstretched there is ipsilateral upward drift or oscillation)
- Hypotonia
- Hyporeflexia.

Causes

- CVA*
  — haemorrhage
  — infarction
- Tumour
  — secondary*
  — primary
  — non-metastatic degeneration (with carcinoma of the bronchus)
- Degenerative
  — multiple sclerosis
  — alcoholism
  — familial, e.g. Friedreich's ataxia
  — hypothyroidism[†].

Note. Lesions of the cerebellar vermis (central part of the cerebellum) cause a peculiar sign called truncal ataxia. This results in instability and writhing movements of the upper torso, accentuated by asking the patient to sit forwards with the arms folded.

ABNORMAL MOVEMENTS

Tremor

Resting

- Physiological* (worse with alcohol)
- Parkinson's disease*
- Benign essential tremor (better with alcohol, often familial)
- Wilson's disease.

Note. Treatment with β_2 agonists and thyrotoxicosis cause an exaggerated physiological tremor.

Worse on movement

- Cerebellar tremor (intention tremor).

Note. Severe Parkinsonian and benign essential tremors are sometimes worse on movement.

Chorea

Sudden, rapid, involuntary and purposeless jerks or fragments of movements. The patient appears fidgety. It is usually a sign of extrapyramidal disease.

Causes

- Drugs, e.g. L-dopa
- CVA (basal ganglia)
- Tumour (basal ganglia)
- Sydenham's chorea
- Thyrotoxicosis
- SLE.

Athetosis

Slow, writhing, sinuous movements. Extrapyramidal.

Causes

- Cerebral palsy*
- Post-cerebral anoxia (e.g. cardiac arrest, drowning, etc.)
- Wilson's disease
- Hereditary.

Hemiballismus[†]

Wild flinging movements in upper limb, due to an ipsilateral lesion to subthalamic nucleus. Responds to chlorpromazine.

DIFFUSE NEUROLOGICAL DISEASE

Many neurological diseases cut across artificial anatomical boundaries. Be prepared to ask to examine other aspects of the nervous system, if you think this is relevant.

CVA*

This causes a pyramidal weakness in both the upper and lower limbs, if the lesion involves the cerebral cortex, internal capsule, or pyramidal tracts as they run through the brain stem. It is important to know the classic distribution of a pyramidal motor weakness.

The weak muscle groups are:

- shoulder abduction
- elbow and wrist extension
- finger abduction
- hip flexors
- hamstrings
- dorsiflexion of foot.

The easy way to remember this is to recall the typical posture of a stroke victim, due to the stronger, intact (spastic) muscle groups. The arm is adducted at the shoulder and flexed at the elbow and wrist. The leg is held straight and the foot drags on walking, due to intact glutei, quadriceps and plantarflexors.

If you find a pyramidal weakness in one leg, it is important to examine the ipsilateral arm and contralateral leg for signs of pyramidal weakness. This is because the causes of a spastic hemiparesis and a spastic paraparesis are quite different (see p. 100).

Multiple sclerosis*

This is a diffuse demyelinating process of unknown aetiology. It commonly starts in early adult life and affects women more frequently than men. It seems to be more common in temperate zones. Spontaneous relapses and remissions occur, but there is usually a gradual overall deterioration through the years. Patients commonly end up wheelchair-bound in the later stages of the disease. The signs will depend on the sites involved and the stage of the disease:

- UMN deficit
  — hemiparesis
  — paraparesis
  — monoparesis
- cerebellar signs
  — often bilateral
  — ataxic nystagmus (pathognomonic)
- optic atrophy

- sensory disturbances
- III, IV or VI nerve palsies
- painless retention of urine
- cerebral cortex involvement — inappropriate euphoria is frequently seen in the later stages of the disease, due to frontal lobe demyelination.

Motor neurone disease

Exceptionally rare in clinical practice. Not quite so rare in exams. There is a progressive, idiopathic degeneration of the anterior horn cells (spinal cord), cranial nerve nuclei and pyramidal tracts. There are *no* sensory signs. There are three patterns of neurological signs, but there is often overlap between these groups:

1. *True bulbar palsy* (see p. 87) — bilateral cranial nerve palsies of IX–XII.
2. *Progressive muscular atrophy* — bilateral degeneration of the anterior horn cells. This causes bilateral lower motor neurone signs in the hands, followed by the feet. There is prominent muscle fasciculation. Loss of deep tendon reflexes.
3. *Amyotrophic lateral sclerosis* — pyramidal tract degeneration; spastic paraparesis. Arms are usually affected later (and less extensively).

Syringomyelia†

Cyst in cervical spinal cord (anterior position). It presents in early adult life and slowly progresses over 20 years. The cyst encroaches on tracts which lie anteriorly:

- lateral spinothalamic (pain and temperature)
- anterior horn cells (LMN)
- pyramidal (UMN).

Signs

- Dissociated sensory loss (arms)
- Painless lesions in the upper limbs
- Charcot's joints (wrist, elbow)
- Wasting of the small muscles of the hand
- UMN signs in the legs.

Syringobulbia[†]

Same as syringomyelia, but the lesion is in the lower brain stem/upper cervical cord. The signs are very similar, but in addition there may be:

- ipsilateral V nerve palsy ⎱ involvement of cranial
- bulbar palsy ⎰ nerve nuclei
- ipsilateral Horner's syndrome (cervical sympathetic nerves)
- nystagmus (brain stem cerebellar connections).

KEY QUESTIONS

Neurology

1. **What are the causes of:**
   - ptosis
   - VI nerve palsy
   - XII nerve palsy
   - pseudobulbar palsy
   - anosmia
   - wasting of the hand
   - carpal tunnel syndrome
   - proximal myopathy
   - parkinsonism
   - sensory neuropathy
   - spastic paraparesis
   - dorsal column loss
   - cerebellar disease
   - resting tremor?
2. **Which muscles of the hand are served by the median nerve?**
3. **What are the causes of an absent red reflex?**
4. **What is Romberg's sign? What is its significance?**
5. **What are the neurological manifestations of the acquired immune deficiency syndrome?**
6. **What is the difference, on clinical examination, between an ulnar nerve palsy and a T1 root lesion?**

2.8

Rheumatology

Rheumatological cases are common in the Final MB because rheumatological disease is common, often resulting in chronic physical signs.

Scheme for examination of the joints

Look — Feel — Move

Inspection

General.   Start by observing the patient generally. Active attention to this point may give you the diagnosis immediately, e.g.:

* butterfly rash on face (SLE)
* small mouth, beaked nosed (scleroderma)
* stooped posture (ankylosing spondylitis)
* scaly rash (psoriatic arthropathy).

Joints.   Now concentrate on the joint(s) in question. The examiner will tell you which joint(s) you are to examine. Look at the joints from the front, back and sides. In particular you are looking for:

* swelling
* erythema
* joint deformity
* scars (previous surgery).

Palpation

Always ask the patient if the joint(s) are tender — if they are, you must palpate carefully. Try not to hurt the patient (keep glancing at the patient's face). Look for:

* tenderness
* synovial thickening

- joint effusion
- deformity
- associated muscle wasting.

Movement

Passive.   Move the patient's joint (gently) to assess its range in all directions of normal movement. Again, be careful, as it is easy to hurt the patient.

Active.   Now ask the patient to move the joint in the same modalities.

Functional movement.   Try to get an idea of how the patient's joint disease has affected that joint's function, e.g.:

- hip joint
  — ask the patient to walk, stand from the sitting position
- hand
  — grip
  — thumb opposition
  — writing
  — use of knife and fork
  — buttoning a shirt, etc.

Further aspects of examination

As directed by your findings. Always look for rheumatoid nodules on the elbows. Also look for:

- nail changes ⎫ psoriatic
- skin lesions ⎬ arthropathy
- gouty tophi (ear, periarticular)
- scleroderma facies/skin
- nailfold telangiectasia (SLE, RA)
- butterfly rash (SLE).

TYPICAL CASES

Rheumatology

- Rheumatoid arthritis
- Systemic lupus erythematosus
- Scleroderma

- Ankylosing spondylitis
- Psoriatic arthropathy
- Monoarthritis
- Raynaud's phenomenon

Rheumatoid arthritis (RA)*

Most commonly you are presented with a pair of arthritic hands. Often, with end-stage disease, the diagnosis is obvious (Fig. 2.8.1). Occasionally you are presented with more acute joints. This is more difficult. The diagnosis may not be immediately obvious, and there is a risk of hurting the patient. If the skin overlying a joint is erythematous, proceed with caution.

Signs

- Hands
  - swelling
  - erythema
  - synovial thickening/tenderness
  - wasting of the small muscles of the hand ⎫
  - deformity, e.g. metacarpophalangeal ⎬ see Fig. 2.8.1
    subluxation ⎭
  - ulnar deviation
  - swan neck deformity ⎫ see Fig. 2.8.2
  - boutonnière deformity ⎭
  - 'Z' deformity of the thumb
  - reduced function
- Always look for rheumatoid nodules (Fig. 2.8.3)
- Ask about other affected joints.

Rheumatoid arthritis usually, but not always, affects joints symmetrically. In the hand, the proximal joints, e.g. the metacarpophalangeal joints (MCP) and the proximal interphalangeal (PIP) joints, are predominantly affected. RA is much more common in females.

Complications of RA

RA is a systemic disease and the complications include:

- Sjögren's syndrome
  - dry eyes
  - dry mouth
  - arthritis

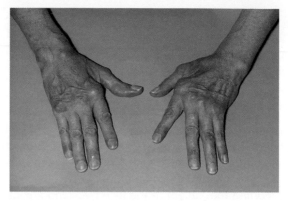

Fig. 2.8.1 Rheumatoid arthritis. Note the prominent metacarpal heads (metacarpophalangeal subluxation), ulnar deviation of the fingers and wasting of the small muscles of the hand.

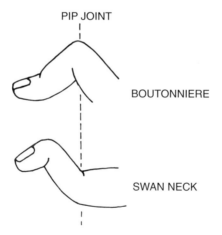

Fig. 2.8.2 Finger deformities: rheumatoid arthritis.

- episcleritis
- fibrosing alveolitis
- Caplan's syndrome (rheumatoid lung nodules with associated pneumoconiosis)
- pericarditis
- vasculitis (vasculitic leg ulcers and mononeuritis multiplex)
- sensory neuropathy

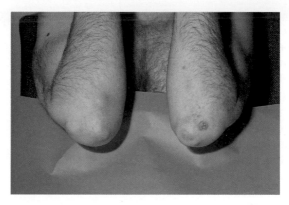

Fig. 2.8.3 Rheumatoid nodules at the elbows.

- Felty's syndrome
  — RA
  — splenomegaly
  — pancytopenia
- amyloidosis (causes renal failure)
- anaemia (of chronic disorders).

Systemic lupus erythematosus

Much more common in women. Onset in early 20s.

Signs

- Arthritis
  — usually symmetrical, often migratory
  — affects the hands, wrists, elbows, knees and ankles
- Skin
  — photosensitivity
  — butterfly rash
  — Raynaud's phenomenon
  — arteritic lesions
  — alopecia
- Sjögren's syndrome
- Lung
  — alveolitis (crackles both sides)
  — pleural effusion

- Heart
  — pericarditis (rub)
  — myocarditis
  — Libman–Sacks endocarditis (right-sided valves involved)
- Kidneys
  — proteinuria
  — nephrotic syndrome
  — chronic renal failure
- Nervous system
  — cerebral lupus
    — confusion
    — intellectual impairment
    — psychiatric symptoms
  — mononeuritis multiplex
  — peripheral neuropathy.

Scleroderma

More common in females.

Signs

- Skin
  — tightened skin which is shiny, with loss of hair and pigmentation. (Try to pick up the skin on the back of the patient's hand between your thumb and index finger. This will be impossible.)
  — telangiectasia
  — facial appearance
    — tight skin
    — beaked nose
    — microstomia
  — Raynaud's phenomenon.
- Chest
  — alveolitis (basal crackles).
- Heart
  — pericarditis (rub)
  — congestive cardiac failure
  — conduction defects.
- Gut
  — oesophageal involvement (dysphagia)
  — small bowel involvement (malabsorption).

- Arthritis
  - small joints of the hand (usually).
- Renal
  - chronic renal failure ± hypertension.

Ankylosing spondylitis

Much more common in men. It usually presents in the 20s or 30s. Over 95% are HLA B27-positive.

Signs

- Fixed spine
  - thoracic kyphosis, loss of lumbar lordosis
  - hyperextension of neck (this results in the typical 'question mark' posture; see Fig. 2.8.4)
- Arthritis
  - large joint monoarthritis of the lower limb
  - sacroiliitis (pelvis 'spring').

X-ray

- Poor chest expansion
- Bamboo spine
- Sacroiliitis.

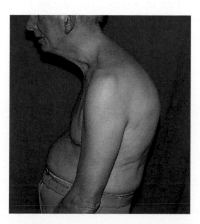

Fig. 2.8.4 The typical 'question mark' posture of ankylosing spondylitis.

Associations

- Aortic regurgitation
- Iritis, conjunctivitis
- Pulmonary fibrosis (apical)
- Mycetoma[†] (fungus ball in under-aerated upper lobe).

Sacroiliitis may also be found in inflammatory bowel disease.

Psoriatic arthropathy

Affects men and women equally.

Signs

- Arthritis (there are three main patterns of joint involvement)
  — *terminal* interphalangeal joints (distinguishes it from RA), usually asymmetrical
  — *polyarthropathy* indistinguishable from RA, but seronegative
  — *arthritis mutilans*: resorption of phalangeal heads resulting in a destructive arthropathy of the hands
- Skin
  — psoriatic plaques
  — pitting of fingernails
  — onycholysis
  — scaling of scalp.

There are no rheumatoid nodules as this is a seronegative arthritis. The skin changes may be minimal, but patients will almost invariably have psoriatic nail changes. Remember that RA and psoriasis are common; not every patient with arthritis and psoriasis will have psoriatic arthropathy. These two conditions can coexist (see Figs 2.8.5 and 2.8.6).

Gout

Chronic gout

Chronic elevation of serum urate.

Signs

- Gouty tophi
  — periarticular
  — pinna of ear

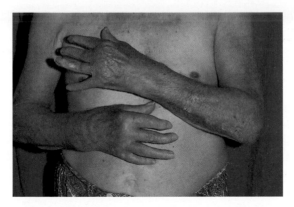

Fig. 2.8.5 Psoriatic arthropathy (arthritis mutilans). Note the patches of psoriasis at the elbows and deformity of the hands, including the distal interphalangeal joints.

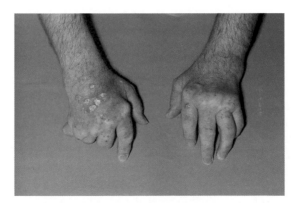

Fig. 2.8.6 Another combination of psoriatic skin lesions and a deforming arthritis of the hands. This time the arthritis is due to rheumatoid arthritis (distal interphalangeal joints relatively spared) and the psoriasis is an incidental finding.

- Arthritis
  — osteoarthrosis (OA) of the affected joints.

Acute gout[†]

Signs

- Arthritis (asymmetrical)
- Great toe

- Wrist/elbow
- Any other joint may be affected.

Causes

- Idiopathic
- Thiazide diuretics
- Renal failure
- Psoriasis
- Myeloproliferative disorders.

Monoarthritis

Causes

- Trauma
- Sepsis
  — bacterial (including tuberculosis and gonorrhoea)
  — viral, e.g. rubella
- Seronegative arthritides
  — osteoarthrosis (OA)
  — psoriasis
  — ankylosing spondylitis (hip, knee)
  — Reiter's disease (ankle, knee)
  — gout
  — pseudogout (knee)
- RA (monoarthritis is an unusual but recognised mode of presentation)
- SLE, scleroderma
- Crohn's disease, ulcerative colitis (hip, knee, ankle).

Raynaud's phenomenon

Signs

- May be none (history important)
- Dystrophic changes
- Loss of the fingertips   } severe cases
- Nail changes   only (see Fig. 2.8.7).
- Frank digital gangrene

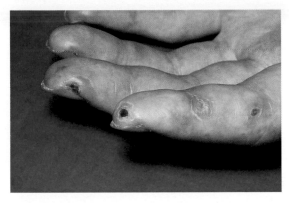

Fig. 2.8.7 Frank digital gangrene in a patient with severe Raynaud's disease.

Causes

- Raynaud's disease (idiopathic)
- Scleroderma
- RA, SLE
- Cervical rib
- Atherosclerotic
- Polycythaemia.

It is more common in people who use vibrating tools. Remember to look for scars in the root of the neck indicating that the patient has had a sympathectomy to alleviate the symptoms.

KEY QUESTIONS

Rheumatology

1. **What are the causes of**
   - Raynaud's phenomenon
   - sacroiliitis
   - gout
   - monoarthritis of the ankle?
2. **What are the differences radiologically between rheumatoid arthritis and osteoarthritis?**
3. **What are the systemic complications of rheumatoid arthritis?**
4. **What is Reiter's syndrome?**

Dermatology

Skin disease is very common but is not examined in detail in the Final MB exam. Candidates are presented with either common dermatological conditions or important dermatological manifestations of systemic disease.

Medical students sometimes believe that dermatological diagnosis is reached through a 'picture matching' process and that the history is irrelevant. This is rarely the case. A logical approach to history and examination is essential. However, if presented with a dermatological case we would recommend an initial brief examination of the skin, as the diagnosis may then be apparent, allowing a more appropriate and relevant history to be taken. In dermatological OSCEs, a logical examination, description of clinical findings, interpretation of physical signs and an appropriate differential diagnosis are much more likely to impress the examiner than the offer of a single diagnosis (which may be incorrect).

Scheme for history of skin conditions

Initial lesion(s)

- Site
- Duration
- Spread
- Exacerbating/relieving factors.

PMH

Associated conditions e.g. atopy in a patient with eczema or immunosuppression (e.g. history of renal transplantation) in a patient with multiple skin cancers.

Drugs

Dermatological side-effects are very common, including from over-the-counter medicines. They may exacerbate pre-existing skin disease. Include previous topical therapy, as this may modify the clinical appearance.

SH

- Environmental factors — occupation and work environment, geographical factors including residence and travel abroad, sun exposure and relevant hobbies
- The impact of the skin condition (physical and psychological) on the patient's life (and that of family) must be assessed.

FH

Many skin conditions have an hereditary component.

Scheme for examination of the skin

Examine the whole skin surface including mouth, eyes and scalp. Ensure optimal lighting — bedside lighting is often inadequate. Look and then palpate. Assess:

- single or multiple lesions
- colour
- surface change — ? scaling
- margin — ill- or well-defined
- temperature
- depth of lesion
- distribution.

Decide whether the pathological process is primarily epidermal (associated with surface change/scaling), dermal or involves the subcutis. For deeper lesions, assess whether they are fixed to under-lying tissues and/or overlying skin.

Consider logically the differential diagnosis and if necessary apply broad categories: inherited, metabolic (rare with skin disease), inflammatory, infection, malignant disease (primary or secondary), drugs, etc.

The distribution of lesions may be extremely helpful in reaching a differential diagnosis. For example, consider external influences (including infection) if the condition appears asymmetrical. Remember, however, that naevoid lesions and blood vessel/lymphatic processes may also result in asymmetrical lesions. Think about ultraviolet radiation, including sunlight, if lesions are confined to exposed skin.

Descriptive terms

- Macule — flat lesion
- Papule — circumscribed raised lesion <1 cm diameter
- Nodule — circumscribed raised lesion >1 cm diameter
- Vesicle, bulla — fluid-filled lesion
- Pustule — pus-filled lesion.

TYPICAL CASES

Dermatology

- Psoriasis
- Dermatitis
- Lichen planus
- Bullous disorders
- Erythema nodosum
- Generalised hyperpigmentation
- Leg ulceration
- Malignant disease

Psoriasis

Very common. Look for:

- well defined scaly plaques (Fig. 2.9.1)
- guttate lesions
- evidence of the Koebner phenomenon (lesions induced by trauma; Fig. 2.9.1)
- nail changes (pitting and onycholysis)
- scalp involvement
- arthropathy.

Pustular psoriasis may be localised to hands and feet or generalised (Fig. 2.9.2). Ask about:

- exacerbating factors — sore throats (streptococcal infection)
- life events and stress

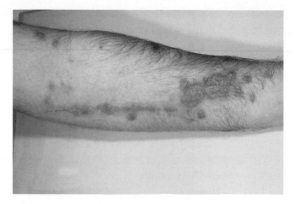

Fig. 2.9.1 Stable plaque psoriasis on forearm. Note linear lesion induced by local trauma (Koebner phenomenon).

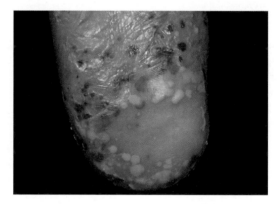

Fig. 2.9.2 Pustular psoriasis of feet. May also be generalised.

- skin trauma, including sunburn
- FH
- previous therapy.

Dermatitis

The terms eczema and dematitis are used interchangeably. May be due to atopic eczema, contact dermatitis, seborrhoeic dermatitis or varicose eczema (see below).

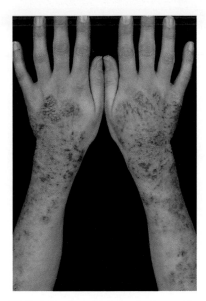

Fig. 2.9.3 Symmetrical ill-defined rash of atopic dermatitis persisting into adult life. Note that flexural involvement is not always seen.

Atopic eczema

Very common. Onset often in early childhood but may persist into adulthood in more severe cases. Widespread, symmetrical ill-defined areas of itchy red papulo-vesicles (Fig. 2.9.3), involving particularly the flexural aspects of elbows and knees. Flexural involvement may not be present, particularly in children less than 1 year old and adults. Xerosis and lichenification may be prominent.

Look for signs of topical steroid overusage, including epidermal atrophy, telangiectasia and striae. Ask about:

- PH or FH of atopy
- exacerbating factors
- details of therapy, including quantities of topical steroids used.

Contact dermatitis

Uncommon in the exam. May be irritant or allergic in nature. Consider this diagnosis when 'eczema' is localised or asymmetrical (Fig. 2.9.4). Remember that allergic contact dermatitis can rarely occur on top of atopic eczema.

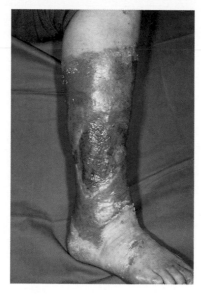

Fig. 2.9.4 Localised allergic contact dermatitis on right lower leg of a patient with venous ulceration. Note the sharp cut-off. Patch-testing demonstrated allergy to parabens, one of the components of medicated bandages.

Ask about:

- occupation
- hobbies
- topical medicaments (Fig. 2.9.4).

Recommend patch testing if allergic contact dermatitis is suspected.

Seborrhoeic dermatitis (Fig. 2.9.5)

Mild disease is common, but if severe consider HIV disease.

Varicose eczema

Always consider whether allergic contact dermatitis contributes to the clinical picture.

Lichen planus

Uncommon. Grouped, very itchy, violaceous flat-topped papules with white interlacing surface (Wickham's striae).

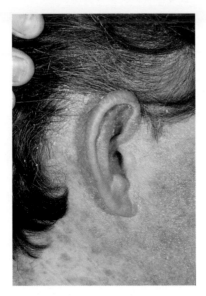

Fig. 2.9.5 Seborrhoeic dermatitis with scaling of the scalp and erythematous scaly rash of face, chest and back.

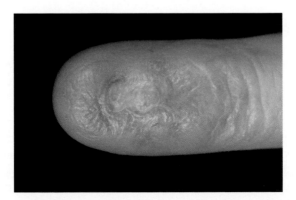

Fig. 2.9.6 Severe scarring and atrophy of nail in a patient with lichen planus. Note fusion of cuticle and nail bed (pterygium formation).

Look for:

- nail changes — pterygium formation (Fig. 2.9.6)
- mucosal changes
- Koebner phenomenon.

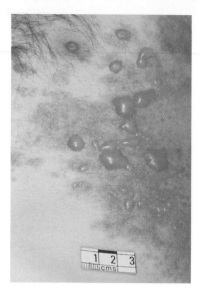

Fig. 2.9.7 Tense intact blisters on an erythematous base in bullous pemphigoid.

Bullous disorders

Rare.

Pemphigoid

Subepidermal tense intact blisters on an inflammatory and often urticated base (Fig. 2.9.7). Age onset 65–75 years. Mucous membrane involvement is uncommon. Histology shows subepidermal bullae with an inflammatory infiltrate including eosinophils. Direct immunofluorescence shows deposition of IgG and C3, along the basement membrane zone.

Pemphigus vulgaris

Intra-epidermal flaccid or deroofed blisters. Age onset 40–60 years. Mucous membrane involvement very common. Histology shows intra-epidermal bullae. Direct immunofluorescence shows deposition of IgG and C3 within the epidermis at keratinocyte junctions.

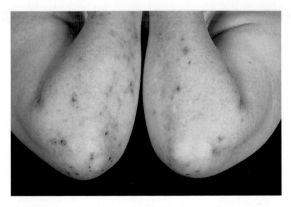

Fig. 2.9.8 Blisters are rarely seen in dermatitis herpetiformis. Note grouped excoriated papules over extensor aspect of elbow.

Dermatitis herpetiformis

Small, very itchy subepidermal blisters on extensor surfaces, particularly elbows, knees and buttocks — often excoriated (Fig. 2.9.8). Age of onset 20–55 years. Associated with gluten-sensitive enteropathy. Direct immunofluorescence shows deposition of IgA at the basement membrane zone.

Other causes of blisters

- Congenital (epidermolysis bullosa)
- Trauma
- Insect bite reaction
- Infections (staphylococcal scalded skin syndrome)
- Photosensitivity
- Drugs (barbiturates)
- Erythema multiforme
- Toxic epidermal necrolysis (TEN).

Erythema nodosum

Uncommon.

Causes

- Infections
  - — streptococcal
  - — TB

- Sarcoidosis
- Inflammatory bowel disease
- Drugs (sulphonamides).

Generalised hyperpigmentation

Uncommon.

Causes

- Addison's disease
- Malabsorption
- Haemochromatosis
- Drugs (chlorpromazine).

Leg ulceration

Very common.

Causes

- Venous (see Fig. 2.9.4)
- Arterial
- Diabetic
- Vasculitis (rheumatoid arthritis)
- Malignant
- Pyoderma gangrenosum
- Sickle cell disease
- Necrobiosis lipoidica.
- Infection (e.g. cellulitis)

Ask about:

- intermittent claudication
- PH of DVT.

Assess:

- edge of ulcer
- distribution of ulcers (venous ulcers generally occur over medial and lateral malleoli)
- arterial system — peripheral pulses
- venous system — varicose veins
- sensation — neuropathic ulcers
- skin — varicose eczema.

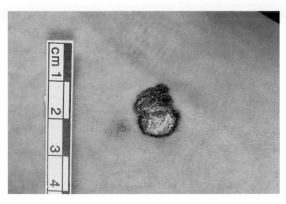

Fig. 2.9.9 Malignant melanoma. Note irregular margin, asymmetry, nodularity, surface change and irregular distribution of pigment.

Look for clues elsewhere (rheumatoid hands, for example). Necrobiosis lipoidica and pretibial myxoedema are covered in Chapter 2.10.

Malignant disease

May be primary or secondary.

Malignant melanoma (Fig. 2.9.9)

Uncommon, but may come up as a clinical slide. Distinguishing clinical features from a benign pigmented lesion are:

- History
  - — changing size
  - — changing colour
  - — changing shape
  - — itching
  - — bleeding
- Examination (Fig. 2.9.9)
  - — diameter >7 mm
  - — irregular outline
  - — asymmetry
  - — irregular distribution of pigment
  - — loss of normal surface markings
  - — oozing/crusting/bleeding/ulceration
  - — raised nodules.

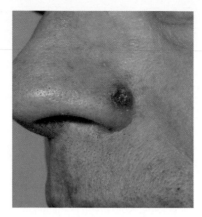

Fig. 2.9.10 Basal cell carcinoma in a characteristic site. Note raised pearly edge.

Basal cell carcinoma

- Common
- Raised nodules with pearly edge and overlying telangiectasia (Fig. 2.9.10)
- No precursor lesions
- Locally invasive but very rarely metastasise.

Squamous cell carcinoma

- Uncommon
- Raised keratinous lesions
- Precursor lesions include Bowen's disease and actinic keratosis
- Metastases are not uncommon.

Cutaneous T-cell lymphoma (mycosis fungoides)

- Rare.
- Well-defined *fixed* scaly plaques.
- Look for associated poikiloderma (telangiectasia, epidermal atrophy and hyperpigmentation).
- May run an indolent course before progressing to tumour stage.
- Systemic involvement and lymphadenopathy are late and often pre-terminal events.
- May result in erythroderma with circulating atypical lymphocytes (Sézary cells). This is very rare.

KEY QUESTIONS

Dermatology

1. With which condition is dermatitis herpetiformis associated?
2. What internal disorders may produce generalised pruritus?
3. How may contact dermatitis be distinguished from atopic dermatitis?
4. What are the cutaneous manifestations of internal malignancy?
5. How would you manage an erythrodermic patient?

Upper limb, lower limb and face

You may be asked to examine part of the patient's anatomy, with no specific clues from the examiner as to which system contains the abnormal physical signs. This can wrong-foot the unwary candidate unless you specifically prepare yourself in advance. The three commonest areas asked about are:

- the upper limb
- the lower limb
- the face.

The question may be: 'Examine this patient's hands' or 'Look at this patient's face'.

You will realise that, because of basic anatomical considerations, you will more than likely find the abnormality in the skin, nervous system or joints. Your examination should be tailored accordingly. Remember to inspect carefully. This may tell you where to concentrate your examination, or give you the diagnosis immediately. Don't forget to examine the peripheral pulses when examining the limbs.

QUESTIONS

The upper limb

If you are presented with an upper limb think of:

- skin
- joints
- nervous system.

The more common upper limb short cases are listed in Table 2.10.1. This is followed by some examples for you to consider (Figs 2.10.1–2.10.6). The answers are found towards the end of the chapter.

Table 2.10.1 Common upper limb cases

Skin (Chapter 2.9)	Psoriasis* Eczema* Lichen planus Dermatitis herpetiformis Scleroderma/Raynaud's
Joints (Chapter 2.8)	RA* OA* Psoriatic arthropathy SLE
Nervous system (Chapter 2.7)	Wasted hand* Ulnar nerve lesion Median nerve lesion Tremor
Miscellaneous	Clubbing* Palmar erythema Psoriatic nail changes Dupuytren's contracture Spider naevi

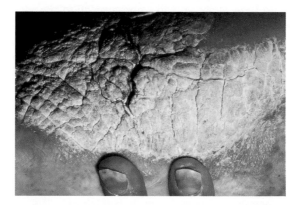

Fig. 2.10.1 (Answer on p. 145)

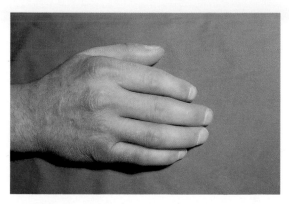

Fig. 2.10.2 (Answer on p. 146)

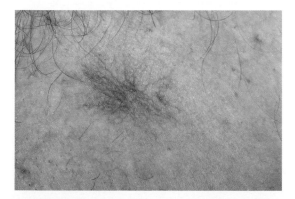

Fig. 2.10.3 (Answer on p. 146)

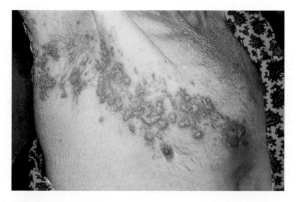

Fig. 2.10.4 (Answer on p. 146)

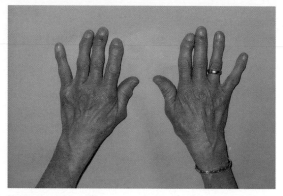

Fig. 2.10.5 (Answer on p. 146)

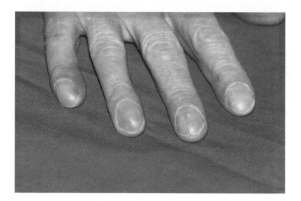

Fig. 2.10.6 (Answer on p. 146)

The lower limb

Again, think of:

- skin
- joints
- nervous system.

Table 2.10.2 lists the more common lower limb cases. Figures 2.10.7–2.10.12 provide examples.

Table 2.10.2 Common lower limb cases	
Skin	Leg ulcers* Psoriasis, dermatitis, etc. Pyoderma gangrenosum[†] Pretibial myxoedema[†] Necrobiosis lipoidica[†]
Joints	RA OA Charcot joint
Nervous system	Peripheral neuropathy* Spastic monoparesis* Spastic paraparesis
Miscellaneous	Bilateral pitting oedema* • CCF • hypoproteinaemia Unilateral swollen leg • cellulitis • DVT • ruptured Baker's cyst Peripheral arterial disease

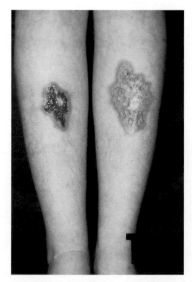

Fig. 2.10.7 (Answer on p. 146)

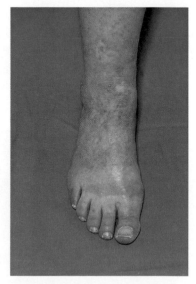

Fig. 2.10.8 (Answer on p. 146)

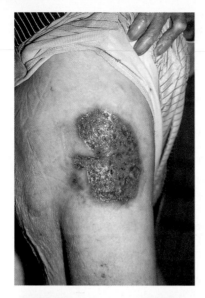

Fig. 2.10.9 (Answer on p. 146)

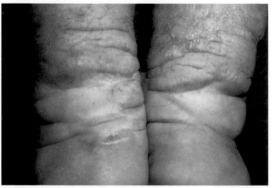

Fig. 2.10.10
(Answer on p. 147)

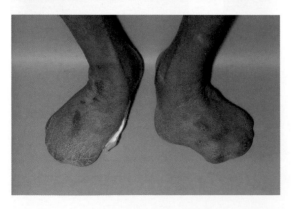

Fig. 2.10.11
(Answer on p. 147)

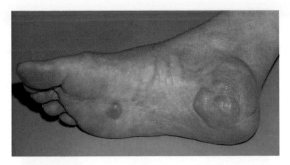

Fig. 2.10.12 (Answer on p. 147)

The face

Rheumatological diseases are less common. Endocrinological disorders are more important. Table 2.10.3 lists common cases. Some examples are given in Figures 2.10.13–2.10.23.

Table 2.10.3 The face: common cases		
Skin	Psoriasis, dermatitis, etc. ⎫ Acne, rosacea ⎬ Chapter 2.9 SLE	Butterfly rash
	Scleroderma	Beaked nose, microstomia
	Herpes zoster	
	Alopecia	
	Xanthelasmata	Hyperlipidaemia
	Lupus pernio	Sarcoid nose
	Dermatomyositis	Heliotrope colour of eyelids
	Hereditary, haemorrhagic telangiectasia	Telangiectasia around mouth
Nervous system	Cranial nerve palsies ⎫ Eye signs ⎬ Chapter 2.7 Parkinsonian facies ⎭	
Endocrine system	Hypothyroidism ⎫ Hyperthyroidism ⎬ See Chapter 2.6 Acromegaly Cushing's syndrome ⎭	
Miscellaneous	Paget's disease	Frontal bossing
	Anaemia ⎫ Jaundice ⎬ See Chapter 2.4	
	Saddle nose	Syphilis, Wegener's granulomatosis

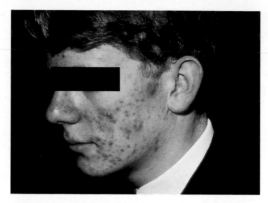

Fig. 2.10.13 (Answer on p. 147)

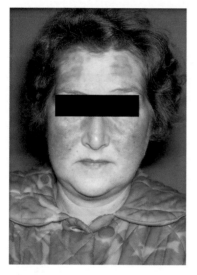

Fig. 2.10.14 (Answer on p. 147)

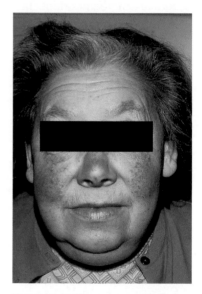

Fig. 2.10.15 (Answer on p. 147)

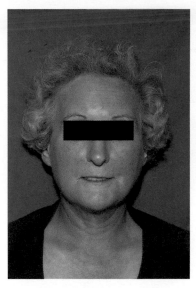

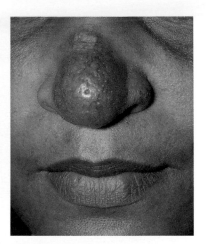

Fig. 2.10.17 (Answer on p. 148)

Fig. 2.10.16 (Answer on p. 147)

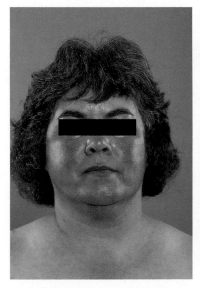

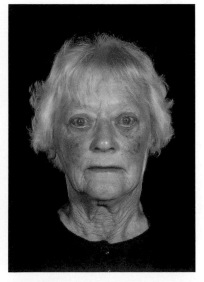

Fig. 2.10.18 (Answer on p. 148)

Fig. 2.10.19 (Answer on p. 148)

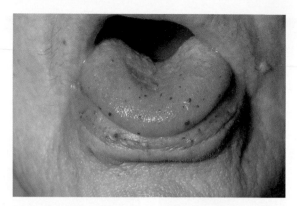

Fig. 2.10.20 (Answer on p. 148)

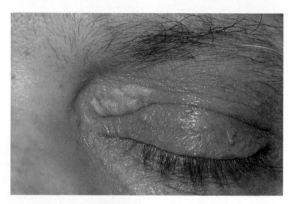

Fig. 2.10.21 (Answer on p. 148)

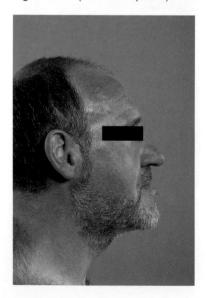

Fig. 2.10.22 (Answer on p. 148)

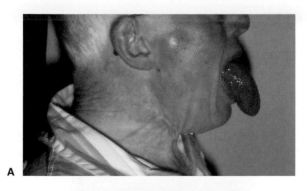

A

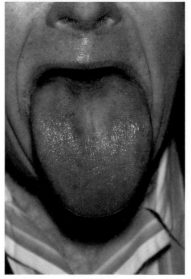

B

Fig. 2.10.23 (Answer on p. 149)

ANSWERS

The upper limb

Figure 2.10.1

This is a case of plaque psoriasis. Note the onycholysis of the nails.

Figure 2.10.2

Scleroderma of hands. The skin on this patient's fingers is puffy, shiny and tethered down. There is some sclerodactyly (tapering of the fingers).

Figure 2.10.3

A spider naevus. These are always found in the area of the body drained by the superior vena cava (upper limb, head, neck and upper trunk). If you find more than three or four, you should look carefully for other signs of chronic liver disease.

Figure 2.10.4

Herpes zoster affecting the T2 dermatome.

Figure 2.10.5

Osteoarthrosis at the terminal interphalangeal joint. Note the Heberden's nodes and the deformity of the distal interphalangeal joint.

Figure 2.10.6

Clubbing of the fingernails.

The lower limb

Figure 2.10.7

Necrobiosis lipoidica. This is a rare complication of diabetes mellitus. Oval indurated plaques found on the shins. Note the brown/yellow margins and yellow waxy areas of atrophy.

Figure 2.10.8

Vitiligo. Very common. Associated with autoimmune conditions such as hypothyroidism, Addison's disease and diabetes mellitus (type 1).

Figure 2.10.9

Pyoderma gangrenosum. It is associated with RA and inflammatory bowel disease. It is found on the lower limb. Note the raised purplish margin and necrotic base. It is very difficult to treat.

Figure 2.10.10

Pretibial myxoedema. Very rare. Pink/skin-coloured induration, areas of which have a 'peau d'orange' appearance. There is sometimes an associated hypertrichosis. Found in thyrotoxicosis.

Figure 2.10.11

This shows some of the complications of diabetes affecting the lower limb. There are bilateral toe amputations (peripheral arterial disease) and Charcot ankle joint (peripheral neuropathy). You can just make out the edge of a dressing on the right: this covers an infected, painless ulcer on the sole of the foot.

Figure 2.10.12

Neurofibromatosis (autosomal dominant). This patient's skin was covered with similar soft subcutaneous and pedunculated tumours. There is an increased incidence of meningioma, glioma and VIII nerve tumours. These benign tumours occasionally undergo sarcomatous change. Also look for café-au-lait patches (>5), scoliosis and unilateral limb hypertrophy.

The face

Figure 2.10.13

Acne vulgaris.

Figure 2.10.14

Butterfly rash of systemic lupus erythematosus.

Figure 2.10.15

Myxoedema. Note the coarse features, 'peaches and cream' complexion and loss of outer third of the eyebrows.

Figure 2.10.16

Scleroderma. Note the tight skin, beaked nose and microstomia. This patient also demonstrates radial furrowing around the lips.

Figure 2.10.17

Lupus pernio. Sarcoidosis of the nose.

Figure 2.10.18

Cushing's syndrome.

Figure 2.10.19

Ophthalmopathy due to Graves' disease. This slide demonstrates true proptosis. (Reproduced by permission from Krentz A J 1997 Colour Guide: Diabetes. Churchill Livingstone, Edinburgh.)

Figure 2.10.20

Hereditary haemorrhagic telangiectasia. Autosomal dominant. These telangiectatic spots are found throughout the upper gastrointestinal tract. The patient usually presents in middle age with recurrent iron deficiency anaemia.

Figure 2.10.21

Xanthelasma.

Fig. 2.10.22

Acromegaly. This patient demonstrates prognathism and has a large nose. The supraorbital ridges are not particularly prominent. Other features to look for include:

- large, burly stature
- spade-like hands and feet
- carpal tunnel syndrome
- organomegaly
- hypertension
- signs of cardiac failure
- bitemporal hemianopia
- large tongue.

Figure 2.10.23

This patient has a huge tongue due to primary amyloidosis. Causes of a large tongue include:

- idiopathic
- carcinoma
- acromegaly
- amyloidosis

PART 3

OSCEs: PRACTICAL SKILLS

Approximately 20–30% of most Final MB OSCE examinations consist of practical skills stations. The range of practical skills which could potentially be assessed is virtually endless. However, the range of practical skills that are commonly tested is much narrower. Think about the day-to-day practical tasks which you will have to perform when you take up your first post after qualification. It is these practical skills that you are most likely to encounter in this section of the examination.

In common with OSCEs testing in other areas of expertise, Final MB practical skills OSCEs are marked using a tick-box approach. It is very important, therefore, to approach the problem and give the answer in a structured and methodical manner.

Have a go at the example below. A model answer, as recorded on the examiner's marksheet, can be found on p. 155.

Q. A 25-year-old female who takes an oestrogen-containing oral contraceptive pill was taken to hospital after suddenly developing dyspnoea and right-sided pleuritic chest pain. On examination there are no physical signs and her CXR and FBC are normal.

- What does the ECG show (Fig. 3.0.1)?
- What is the differential diagnosis?
- What action would you take?

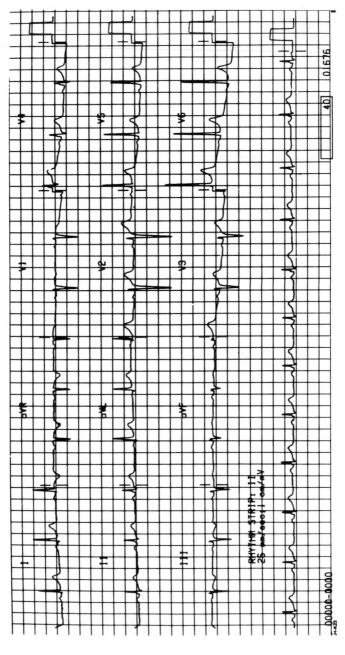

Fig. 3.0.1

Examiners' tick-box answer sheet

	Answer	Possible marks
Rate	75/min	1
Rhythm	Sinus rhythm	1
Axis	0°	1
P wave	Normal	$\frac{1}{2}$
PR interval	0.12 s	$\frac{1}{2}$
QRS complex	Normal	$\frac{1}{2}$
ST segment	Normal	$\frac{1}{2}$
T waves	Normal	$\frac{1}{2}$
U waves	Absent	$\frac{1}{2}$
Pattern recognition	Normal ECG	4
Differential diagnosis	Pulmonary embolus	4
	Musculoskeletal pain	1
Action plan	• Admit to hospital	1
	• Give oxygen	1
	• Blood gases	1
	• Anticoagulate	1
	• CT pulmonary angiography	1
	TOTAL	20

This example may have caused some of you to become anxious. Don't panic and read on.

3.1

The electrocardiogram (ECG)

You need to have a basic grasp of the ECG: you ought to be able to recognise simple abnormalities, e.g. myocardial infarction, ventricular fibrillation/tachycardia, heart block, etc. ECGs and rhythm recognition are taught poorly at many medical schools. This next chapter should help considerably. We have tried to keep it as simple and as understandable as possible.

READING THE ECG

Look at each individual part of the ECG in turn, using the following list:

- rate
- rhythm
- axis
- P wave
- PR interval
- QRS complex
- ST segment
- T wave
- U wave
- pattern recognition.

Like most things in medicine it is best to start off with a routine and adhere rigidly to it, at least in the first instance. Look at as many ECGs as possible and read them using this scheme. You will eventually reach a point (perhaps in years to come) when a glance will be sufficient to tell you the diagnosis (by pattern recognition). Do not do this in the examination.

Note. On most ECGs with standard settings: one small square (1 mm) = 0.04 s; one large square (5 mm) = 0.2 s.

Rate

Simple. Measure the distance (in large squares) between two consecutive R waves and divide into 300, that is:

$$\frac{300}{R - R \text{ interval}}$$

For example, if the R − R interval is four large squares:

$$\text{Rate} = \frac{300}{4} = 75 \text{ beats/min}$$

Bradycardia: rate < 60; tachycardia: rate > 100.

Rhythm

This can be rather more tricky. Having said this, we think it would be unfair for you to be shown a complex arrhythmia.

Normal sinus rhythm

There is a P wave before each QRS complex.

- PR interval < 0.2 s (five small squares).
- QRS complex width < 0.12 s (three small squares).

Ectopics (Fig. 3.1.1)

- Ventricular. The QRS complex is wide (<0.12 s) and bizarre in shape.
- Atrial. The P wave is an unusual shape, or may be inverted. It will come slightly earlier or slightly later than expected. The QRS complex is normal width.

Tachyarrhythmias

Supraventricular. The width of the QRS complex is normal (i.e. <0.12 s) and the rate >100 beats/min.

- Sinus tachycardia. P wave before each QRS complex. R − R interval regular.
- Supraventricular tachycardia. P waves may not be evident, e.g. nodal tachycardia, atrial tachycardia. Regular R − R interval.
- Atrial fibrillation. No P waves. Irregularly irregular R − R interval. Irregular fibrillating pattern of baseline.

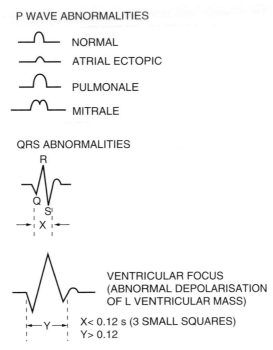

P WAVE ABNORMALITIES

NORMAL

ATRIAL ECTOPIC

PULMONALE

MITRALE

QRS ABNORMALITIES

R

Q

S

X

VENTRICULAR FOCUS
(ABNORMAL DEPOLARISATION
OF L VENTRICULAR MASS)

Y

X< 0.12 s (3 SMALL SQUARES)
Y> 0.12

Fig. 3.1.1 P wave and QRS abnormalities.

Ventricular

- Ventricular tachycardia (VT). Broad complex (QRS > 0.12 s). Tachyarrhythmia (rate > 100 beats/min). P wave impossible to see (usually).

Occasionally atrial beats can be conducted to the ventricles through an abnormal pathway at the a-v node. This can cause an SVT with aberrant conduction, which may be indistinguishable from VT. (This is postgraduate medicine.)

- Ventricular fibrillation (VF). Bizarre waveform with no discernible baseline or meaningful complexes. The patient will have no output ('cardiac arrest'). If the patient has a pulse then check the ECG leads, as one has probably fallen off.

Bradyarrhythmias

Sinus bradycardia. P waves are present and regular. Rate < 60 beats/min. Normal QRS configuration.

Nodal. No P waves at all. Rate < 60 beats/min. Normal QRS configuration.

Heart block (Fig 3.1.2). This is caused by an increased refractory period of the a-v node (of varying degrees of severity). In complete heart block the a-v node will allow no electrical impulse to pass from the atria to the ventricles, which therefore function independently.

- First degree (1°). PR interval > 0.2 s. All P waves followed by normal QRS.

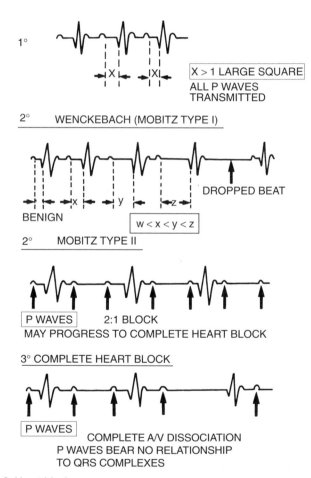

Fig. 3.1.2 Heart block.

- Second degree (2°)
  Wenckebach (Mobitz type I). PR interval gradually increases in length until there is a dropped beat (atrial beat not transmitted to ventricles via a-v node).
  Mobitz type II. PR interval 0.2 s. Dropped beats (a-v conduction failure) are regular: e.g. two to one block (2:1) — alternate beats dropped; three to one block (3:1) — every third beat dropped. Mobitz type II has a more serious prognosis, as it often progresses to complete heart block.

- Complete heart block (3°).   Complete a-v dissociation. P waves bear no relationship to QRS. QRS may be wide and bizarrely shaped. The rate may drop to a very low value (20 beats/min). This causes reduced cardiac output and syncope.

Axis

Easy, if you know how. Use the diagram of electrical vectors (Fig. 3.1.3) and the standard leads (I, II, III, AVF, AVL, AVR) of the ECG in Figure 3.0.1 (p. 154).

Find the *isoelectric lead* (i.e. the one in which the size of the R wave is most equivalent to the size of the S wave). In this case it is lead AVF. Check this against the diagram of electrical vectors (Fig. 3.1.3). In this instance the isoelectric vector will be at approximately

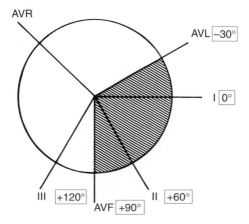

Fig. 3.1.3 Electrical axis. The shaded area represents the normal range of electrical axis.

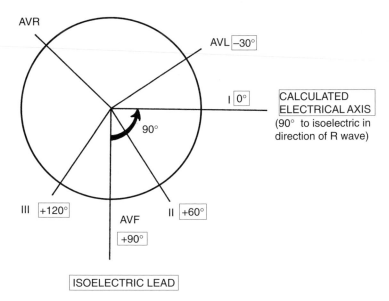

Fig. 3.1.4 Working out the electrical axis. The calculation of electrical axis in this diagram refers to the ECG in Figure 3.0.1 (p. 154).

+90°. Now look at the ECG again and find the lead(s) with the greatest positive deflection (i.e. the largest R waves). In this case, this is I and AVL.

The electrical axis of the heart will be at 90° to the isoelectric lead in the direction of the large R waves: electrical axis = 0°; normal axis ranges from +90° to −30° (see Fig. 3.1.4).

P wave (Fig. 3.1.1)

It should be less than 2.5 mm tall. It is tallest in lead II and it is for this reason that lead II is often used as the rhythm strip:

- 'P' mitrale (mitral valve disease) — double-topped P wave due to left atrial enlargement
- 'P' pulmonale (pulmonary hypertension) — large single-peaked P wave due to right atrial enlargement.

PR interval

From the start of the P wave to the start of the R wave should be 0.12–0.2 s (three to five small squares):

- PR > 0.2 s = first-degree heart blocks
- PR < 0.12 s is seen in the re-entrant tachycardias, e.g. Wolff–Parkinson–White syndrome.

QRS complex

Q waves

Q waves are normally seen in AVR. They are sometimes seen in III in normal individuals. Pathological Q waves are greater than 1 mm × 1 mm and denote transmural infraction of the myocardium.

R waves

The R wave should get bigger as you go across the V leads, V1–6. There is often little or no R wave in V1.
Causes of large R wave in V1 are:

- dextrocardia
- pulmonary embolus
- right ventricular hypertrophy
- Wolff–Parkinson–White (type A)
- true posterior myocardial infarction.

In Wolff–Parkinson–White syndrome (W–P–W) the R wave has a slurred upstroke (delta wave) due to abnormal conduction of impulses through the a-v node via an aberrant pathway (see Fig. 3.1.5). These patients are prone to tachyarrhythmias such as atrial fibrillation.

S wave

The S wave should get smaller as you traverse the V leads (V1–V6).

Bundle branch block (BBB)

Here the QRS complex is wide (>0.12 s). In right BBB the QRS complex will be mainly upright in V1 and V2. In left BBB the QRS complex will be mainly upright in leads V5 and V6. LBBB makes the rest of the ECG uninterpretable (see 'typical cases' pp. 175–176).

ST segment

This should normally be at the same level as the baseline.

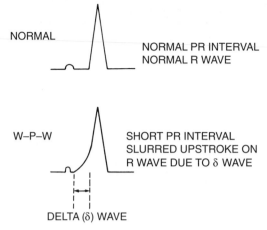

Fig. 3.1.5 The delta wave.

Raised ST segment

* Convex upwards
  — acute myocardial infarction
  — some normal black people
* Concave upwards
  — pericarditis (especially in leads V5, V6, I and AVL).

Depressed ST segment

* Acute myocardial ischaemia
* Digoxin effect (see Fig. 3.1.6)

Note. The 'digoxin effect' does not imply digoxin toxicity, but simply that the patient is currently taking digoxin.

T wave

Peaked T wave

* Myocardial ischaemia
* Hyperkalaemia.

Peaked T waves are occasionally seen in the very early stages of acute myocardial infarction.

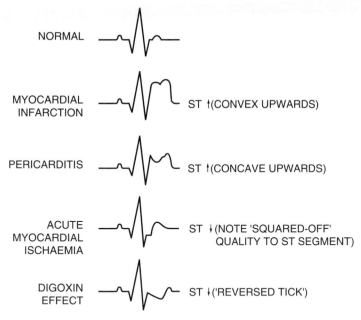

Fig. 3.1.6 Abnormal ST segments.

Inverted T wave

- Myocardial ischaemia
- Post-myocardial infarction
- Hypokalaemia
- Left ventricular hypertrophy/strain
- Following a bundle branch block pattern.

U waves

Seen after the T wave as a little blip on the baseline.

Causes

- Normal fit young adults
- Myocardial ischaemia
- Hypokalaemia.

Pattern recognition

Essentially this means synthesising all the information you have gleaned from going through the above scheme. You should try to fit all the abnormalities together to make a diagnosis.

Experts can glance at an ECG and make an immediate diagnosis. This comes from years of practice perfecting their pattern recognition skills. You may find such people rather irritating — don't worry, you will be able to do it in the end; it's just a matter of enough practice.

TYPICAL CASES

This section gives you a chance to read specimen ECGs, similar to the ones you may be presented with during the examination (Figs 3.1.7–3.1.17). We suggest that you read them in the way we have demonstrated. The answers are to be found on the page following the ECG.

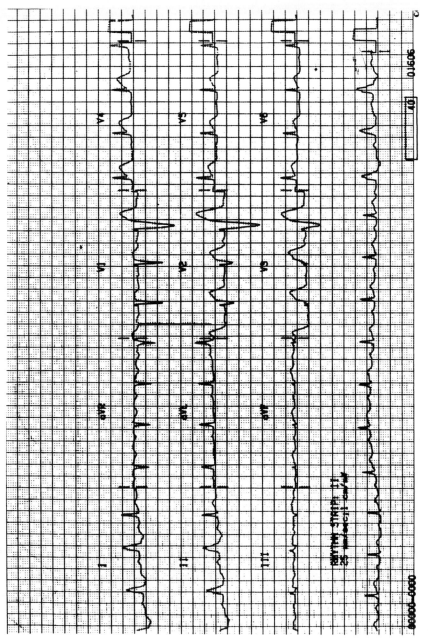

Fig. 3.1.7 Case 1.

Case 1

Rate:	80/min
Rhythm:	Sinus
Axis:	0°
P wave:	Normal
PR interval:	0.2 s (upper limit of normal)
QRS complex:	One ventricular ectopic (V1–3) Broad-looking complexes I, II
ST segment:	Raised V2–6
T wave:	Prominent V2–5
U wave:	Absent
Pattern recognition:	Acute anterior myocardial infarction

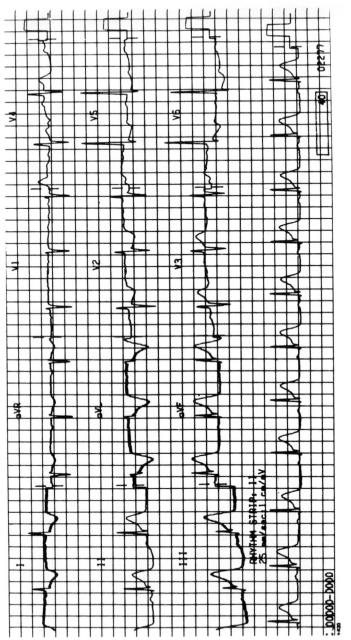

Fig. 3.1.8 Case 2.

Case 2

Rate:	70/min
Rhythm:	Sinus
Axis:	+60°
P wave:	Normal
PR interval:	0.16 s
QRS complex:	Normal
ST segment:	Raised ST II, III, AVF Depressed ST V5, 6, I, AVL
T wave:	Inverted V4–6, I, AVL
U wave:	Present V4–6
Pattern recognition:	Acute inferior myocardial infarction, with associated anterolateral myocardial ischaemia

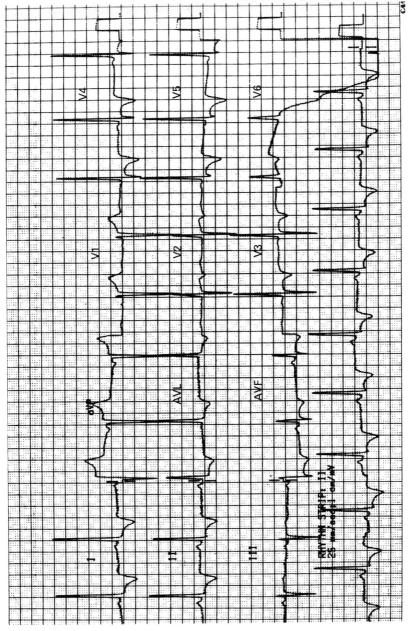

Fig. 3.1.9 Case 3.

Case 3

Rate:	60/min
Rhythm:	Sinus
Axis:	+15°
P wave:	Normal
PR interval:	0.12 s
QRS complex:	Large R waves V2–6, I, II
	Deep S waves V1–3
	R wave V5 + S wave V1 = 49 mm
ST segment:	Widespread depression
T wave:	Inverted V2–6, I, II, AVL, AVF
U wave:	Absent
Pattern recognition:	Left ventricular hypertrophy

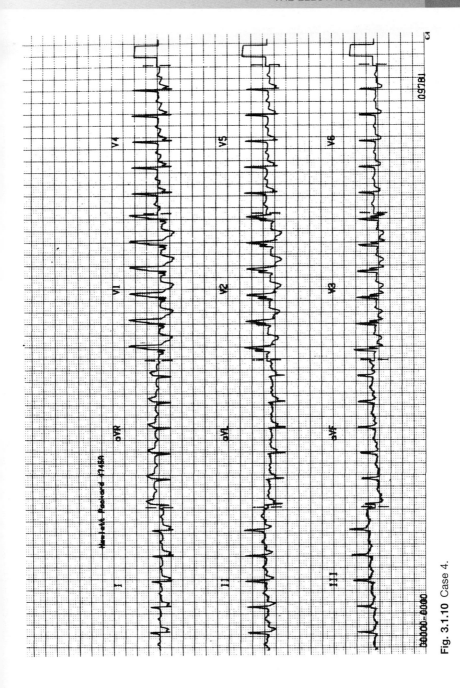

Fig. 3.1.10 Case 4.

Case 4

Rate:	150/min
Rhythm:	Atrial fibrillation
Axis:	+90°
P wave:	Absent
QRS complex:	Wide complexes V1–3 'M' pattern
ST segment:	Depressed V1–3
T wave:	Inverted V1–3
U wave:	Absent
Pattern recognition:	1. RBBB 2. Sinus tachycardia, cause unknown

Note. ST segment and T wave changes are secondary to RBBB.

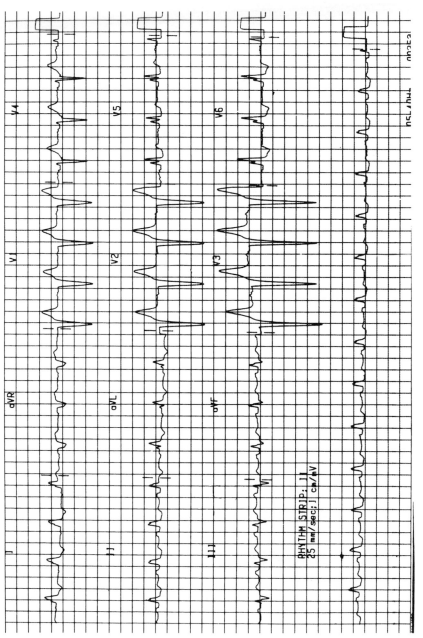

Fig. 3.1.11 Case 5.

Case 5

Rate:	85/min
Rhythm:	Sinus
Axis:	+30°
P wave:	Rather broader than normal
PR interval:	0.16 s
QRS:	Wide Bizarre-looking 'M' pattern V5–6
ST segment:	Depressed I, II, AVF, AVL, V5–6
T waves:	Inverted V5, V6, I, II, AVL
U waves:	Absent
Pattern recognition:	LBBB, aetiology unknown

Note.   The ST segment and T wave abnormalities are secondary to LBBB.

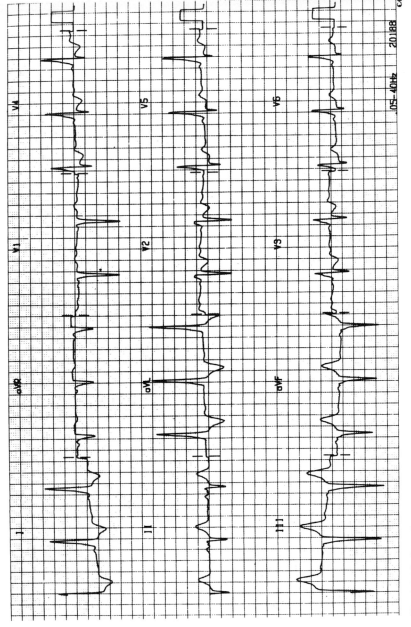

Fig. 3.1.12 Case 6.

Case 6

Rate:	65/min
Rhythm:	Sinus
Axis:	−60° (left axis deviation)
P wave:	Normal
PR interval:	0.1 s (abnormally short)
QRS complex:	Abnormal-looking Width 0.12 s Slurred upstroke to R wave (delta wave)
ST segment:	Depressed V2–6, I, AVL
T wave:	Inverted V2–4, I, AVL
U waves:	Absent
Pattern recognition:	Wolff–Parkinson–White syndrome

Note.   This ECG bears a striking similarity to LBBB (Case 5).

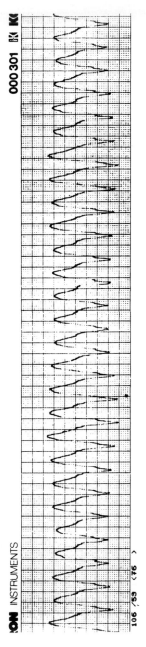

Fig. 3.1.13 Case 7.

Case 7

Broad complex tachycardia.

Rate: 150/min

Diagnosis: Ventricular tachycardia (VT)

This may be impossible to distinguish from SVT with aberrant conduction without doing sophisticated electrophysiological studies (see main text).

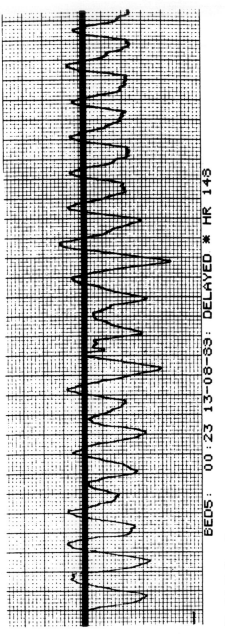

BED5: 00:23 13-08-83: DELAYED * HR 148

Fig. 3.1.14 Case 8.

Case 8

Broad complex trace with no discernible underlying rhythm.

Patient pulseless.

Diagnosis: Ventricular fibrillation (VF)

This patient needs immediate defibrillation.

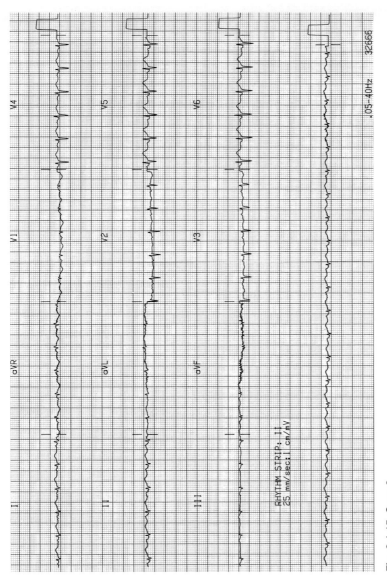

Fig. 3.1.15 Case 9.

Case 9

Rate:	150/min
Rhythm:	Sinus rhythm
Axis:	Difficult to tell!
P wave:	Normal
PR interval:	0.16 s
QRS complex:	Uniformly low voltage throughout
ST segment:	Normal
T wave:	Normal
U wave:	Absent
Pattern recognition:	Pericardial effusion

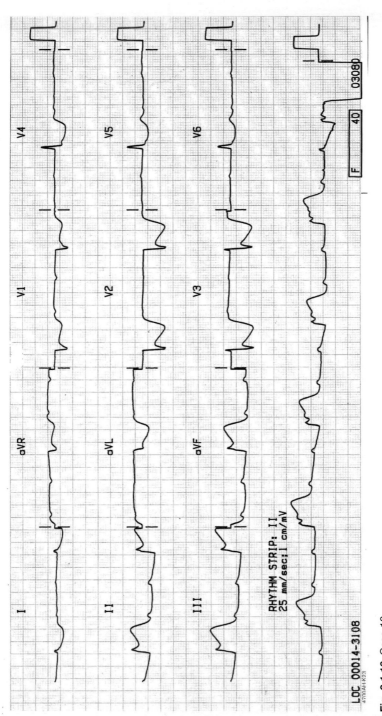

Fig. 3.1.16 Case 10.

Case 10

Rate:	38/min
Rhythm:	Complete heart block (don't be fooled — there are P waves hidden in the ST segments)
Axis:	+90°
P wave:	Normal
PR interval:	Complete dissociation of P waves from QRS complex
QRS complex:	Normal
ST segment:	ST elevation II, III, AVF ST depression I, AVR, AVL, V1–5.
T wave:	See above
U wave:	Absent
Pattern recognition:	Acute inferior myocardial infarction with reciprocal changes and complete heart block.

Note. The inferior territory of the heart is supplied by the right coronary artery, which also supplies the atrioventricular node in 80–90% of people. Bradycardias and complete heart block are much more common after an inferior myocardial infarction.

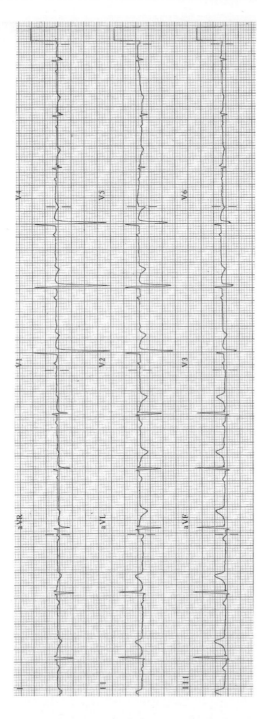

Fig. 3.1.17 Case 11.

Case 11

Rate:	65/min
Rhythm:	Sinus rhythm
Axis:	+120° (right axis deviation)
P wave:	Normal
PR interval:	0.16 s
QRS complex:	Positive R wave V1–2 QRS amplitude diminishes from V1 to V6
ST segment:	Normal
T wave:	Inverted V1–6
U wave:	Absent
Pattern recognition:	Dextrocardia

KEY QUESTIONS

ECG

We have made it easy this time by including the answers.

1. **ECG changes in pulmonary embolus*:**
   - none*
   - sinus tachycardia
   - RBBB
   - S1, Q3, T3[†] (S wave in I, Q wave in III, inverted T in III).

2. **ECG changes in myocardial infarction*:**
   - none
   - hyperacute, peaked T waves
   - ST elevation
   - Q waves
   - T wave inversion.

   These changes occur over the first 36 hours. Q waves and T wave inversion may persist.

3. **Arrhythmias in myocardial infarction*.**

   The answer to this is easy: any (see earlier in this chapter).

4. **Causes of sinus bradycardia*:**
   - vasovagal syncope
   - fit young athletes
   - post-myocardial infarction
   - iatrogenic (β blocker)
   - raised intracranial pressure
   - myxoedema ⎫
   - jaundice ⎬ rare.
   - hypothermia ⎭

5. **Causes of sinus tachycardia*:**
   - anxiety
   - pain
   - post-myocardial infarction
   - iatrogenic (β agonists)
   - pulmonary embolus
   - shock (of any aetiology)
   - thyrotoxicosis
   - fever.

6. **ECG effects of digoxin*:**
   - 'reversed tick' sign (Fig. 3.1.6)
   - a-v block
   - any arrhythmia, but especially electrical bigeminy and paroxysmal atrial tachycardia, with block (digoxin toxicity).
7. **Hypokalaemia*:**
   - prominent U wave
   - inverted T wave
   - ST depression
   - PR prolongation (see Fig. 3.1.18)
8. **Hyperkalaemia*:**
   - tall, peaked T wave
   - QRS widening
   - absent P wave (see Fig. 3.1.18)
9. **The ECG differences between pericarditis and pericardial effusion:**
   - pericarditis — ST elevation (concave upwards) V4–5, I, AVL (Fig. 3.1.6)
   - pericardial effusion — small-voltage ECG in all leads (Fig. 3.1.15).

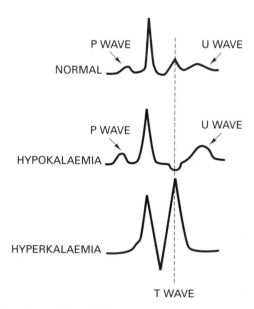

Fig. 3.1.18 Potassium and the ECG.

10. **The ECG criteria for left ventricular hypertrophy (LVH):**
    - tall R waves V5, 6
    - deep S waves V1, 2
      (*Note.* If the height of the R wave in V6 plus the depth of the S wave in V1 is greater than 40 mm, this is definite evidence of LVH.)
    - inverted T waves (sometimes) V4–6
    - LAD.

11. **Causes of left axis deviation (LAD) (axis –30° to –120°):**
    - left anterior hemiblock
    - inferior myocardial infarction
    - chronic obstructive airways disease
    - Wolff–Parkinson–White syndrome
    - left ventricular hypertrophy.

12. **Cause of right axis deviation (RAD) (axis +90° to +180°):**
    - right ventricular hypertrophy
    - dextrocardia
    - Wolff–Parkinson–White syndrome
    - left posterior hemiblock (diagnosed by excluding the others)
    - leads on wrong way round.

13. **Causes of LBBB (always an abnormal finding):**
    - ischaemic heart disease
    - hypertension
    - aortic valve disease
    - following cardiac surgery.

14. **Causes of RBBB:**
    - pulmonary embolism
    - ischaemic heart disease
    - atrial septal defect
    - chronic pulmonary hypertension
    - myocarditis
    - some normal patients.

Radiology

The radiographs you may be asked to comment on during the course of the OSCE will not be complicated or too exotic — this would be unfair.

You need to try to demonstrate several things to the examiner. Firstly, appear as though you are familiar with looking at radiographs. Secondly, show that you have a logical, methodical approach to their interpretation. Finally, demonstrate that you can spot gross abnormalities, even if you are unsure what they represent.

To achieve these aims you need to practise looking at some radiographs, of the kind which crop up in the examination, using a systematic approach to their interpretation.

Approach to the chest radiograph

1. Always view on a well-lit viewing box

2. Look at the side marker (L or R)

This is to make sure that the radiograph has been put up the correct way round. There are several causes of an 'R' marker on the left of a chest radiograph:

- radiograph put on the viewing box the wrong way round
- radiograph marked incorrectly by the radiographer
- dextrocardia.

In the latter two cases the 'R' marker is on the same side as the cardiac apex.

3. Check name and date of birth

They may give important clues.

4. Determine whether the radiograph is a postero-anterior (PA) or anteroposterior (AP)

In PA views the cardiothoracic ratio (ratio of the transverse size of the cardiac outline to the transverse size of the thoracic cage) is normally less than 0.5. An AP projection will cause an apparent increase in this ratio (where none actually exists) because of the way in which the radiograph has been taken. Therefore, you must *never* comment on the cardiothoracic ratio of an AP chest radiograph.

If an AP view has been taken the radiographer should label the film 'AP' (see Case 9). This can be checked by looking at the position of the scapulae on the film. In an AP projection the scapulae overlie the lung fields, but in a good-quality PA view they should not (compare Cases 9 and 10).

5. View the radiograph as a whole

Your eye may be caught by a gross abnormality.

6. View each part of the radiograph in turn

Ignore the temptation to blurt out your first impression. You must now methodically look at each part of the radiograph in turn, to see if you can spot any other abnormalities. We recommend that you use the following scheme:

- soft tissues
  - breasts
  - subcutaneous tissues
    - chest
    - neck
    - arms
- bony structures
  - humeri
  - scapulae
  - clavicles
  - cervical/thoracic spine
  - ribs
- pleura and diaphragm
- mediastinal structures
- lung fields.

7. Take another look at the radiograph as a whole

8. Synthesise

Now synthesise the above steps, to arrive at your answer. Remember to relate the radiological findings to any clinical information you already know about the patient. Try to illustrate to the examiner that you have looked at the radiograph methodically. For example:

Question: 'What abnormalities do you see on this chest radiograph?'

Bad answer (although correct): 'Carcinoma of the bronchus.'

Good answer: 'There is a 4 cm nodule in the mid-zone of the left lung field. This has a slightly irregular margin. The superior edge is particularly indistinct, with linear shadows radiating into the left upper lobe. The most likely cause for this appearance would be carcinoma of the bronchus. I can see no evidence of metastatic spread to the bones, mediastinal structures or other lung field, which all appear normal.'

The 'bad answer' will score considerably worse than the good answer on an OSCE examiner's tick-box sheet. Giving this type of 'bad answer' runs a serious risk of scoring zero if you get the diagnosis wrong. If you adopt the approach of the 'good answer', you will still get a good mark even if you get the diagnosis wrong.

This general approach can be applied to any radiograph, including contrast radiology. Once you have got the general idea, all you need is practice.

SPECIMEN CASES

We have included some radiological cases for you to consider (Figs 3.2.1–3.2.18).

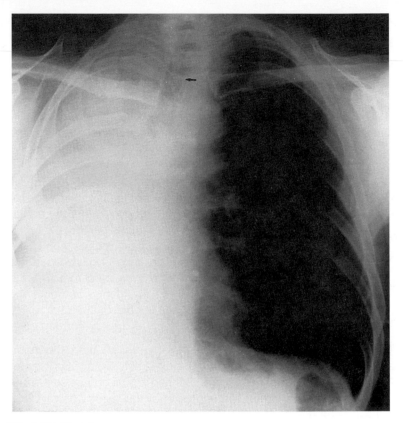

Fig. 3.2.1 Case 1.

This is a PA chest radiograph.
The whole of the right lung field is radio-opaque ('white-out').
The arrow indicates the left margin of the trachea. This,
together with the position of the cardiac outline (which is barely
visible), implies mediastinal shift to the right, due to loss of
lung volume on this side.
The right fifth rib is absent.
Soft tissues — normal.
Conclusion. Post-pneumonectomy chest radiograph.

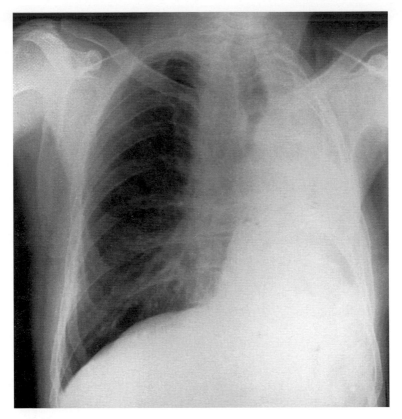

Fig. 3.2.2 Case 2.

This is a PA chest radiograph.
The whole of the left lung field is radio-opaque.
There is considerable loss of volume of the left lung (tracheal and mediastinal deviation to the left).
Bony structures — normal.
Soft tissues — normal.
Conclusion. Collapse, left lung. In this case it was due to a large carcinoma of the bronchus obstructing the left main bronchus. This was confirmed at bronchoscopy.

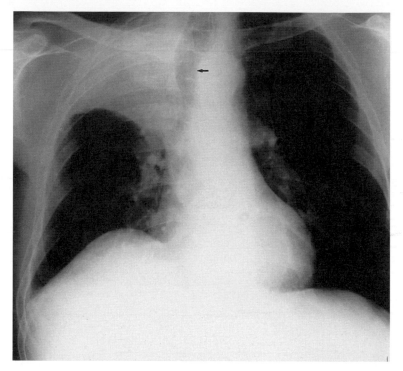

Fig. 3.2.3 Case 3.

This is a PA chest radiograph.
The right lung has a homogeneous radio-opaque area in the upper zone. This has a sharply demarcated lower edge, convex upwards, which is almost certainly an abnormally high horizontal fissure.
The trachea is pulled over to the right.
The right hemidiaphragm is domed medially, and slightly higher than normal.
Bony structures — normal.
Soft tissues — normal.
Conclusion. Partial collapse, right upper lobe.

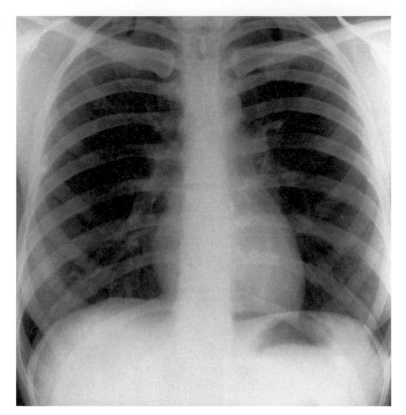

Fig. 3.2.4 Case 4.

This is a normal PA chest radiograph.

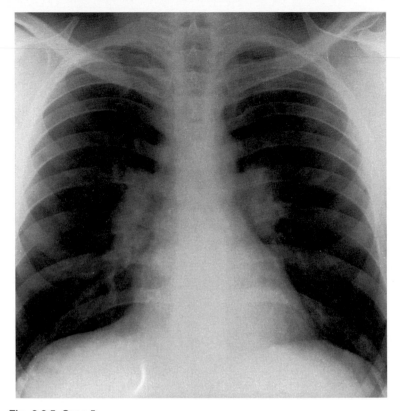

Fig. 3.2.5 Case 5.

This is a PA chest radiograph.
There is bilateral hilar lymphadenopathy.
In addition to this there is also paratracheal lymphadenopathy (look adjacent to the trachea, just below the medial end of the right clavicle).
Lung fields — normal.
Pleura — normal.
Bones — normal.
Soft tissues — normal.
Conclusion. Bilateral hilar lymphadenopathy. Possible causes:

- sarcoidosis
- tuberculosis
- lymphoma.

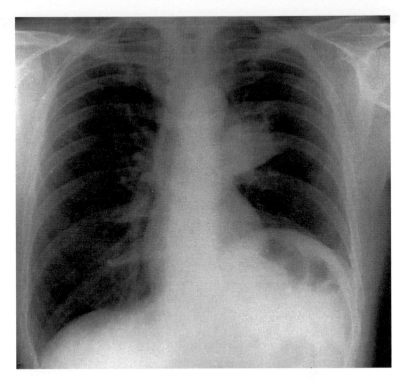

Fig. 3.2.6 Case 6.

This is a PA chest radiograph.
There is a mass at the left hilum. Its inferior surface is well
demarcated, but its superior and lateral edges are irregular.
Its medial surface merges with the mediastinal structures.
There is a raised left hemidiaphragm.
Right lung — normal.
Bony structures — normal.
Soft tissues — normal.
Conclusion. Carcinoma of the bronchus causing a left phrenic
nerve palsy.

The phrenic nerve palsy can be confirmed radiologically by
fluoroscopic screening of the diaphragm.

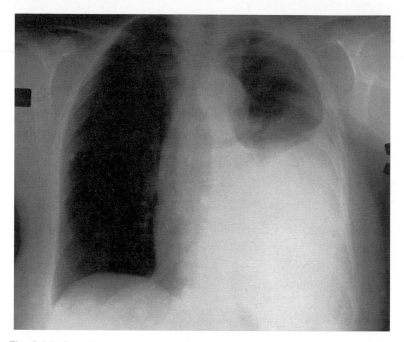

Fig. 3.2.7 Case 7.

This is a PA chest radiograph.
There is homogeneous shadowing in the lower and midzones of the left lung field. The superior border is well demarcated and concave upwards.
The left costophrenic angle has been obscured.
The mediastinum is central.
The right lung field is normal.
The left breast is absent.
Bony structures — normal.
Conclusion. Left pleural effusion.

Subsequent investigation revealed it to be due to metastatic adenocarcinoma. The primary was removed from the left breast 8 years previously.

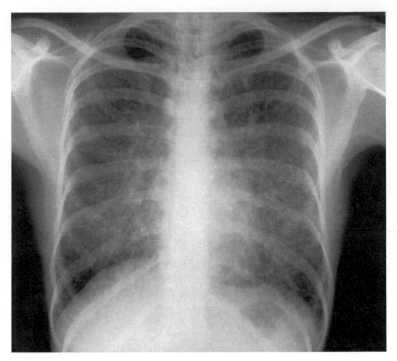

Fig. 3.2.8 Case 8.

This is a PA chest radiograph.

There are small nodules (1–2 cm diameter) and fine line shadows spread evenly throughout both lung fields (reticulonodular shadowing). There is, possibly, relative sparing of the apices.

Mediastinal structures — normal.

Pleura/diaphragm — normal.

Bony structures — normal.

Soft tissues — normal.

Conclusion. Reticulonodular shadowing, cause unknown.

There are many possible causes, including:

- miliary tuberculosis
- sarcoidosis
- pneumoconiosis
- lymphangitis carcinomatosa.

This case was due to sarcoidosis.

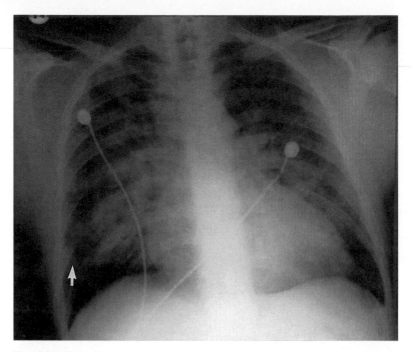

Fig. 3.2.9 Case 9.

This is an AP chest radiograph. Note the position of the medial border of the scapulae, which commonly project over the edge of the lung fields in an AP film.

There is fluffy shadowing in both lung fields, particularly in the mid-zones. The upper lobe vessels are bulky. There are Kerley B lines (arrowed at the right base). ECG leads are present.

Soft tissues — normal.

Pleura and diaphragm — normal.

Bony structures — normal.

Conclusion. Pulmonary oedema.

Note. You cannot comment on the cardiac size on this film, even though it looks large, as it is an AP view.

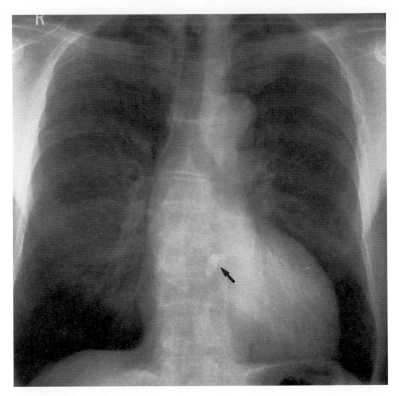

Fig. 3.2.10 Case 10.

This is a PA chest radiograph.
The cardiothoracic ratio is 0.52, which is just above the normal limit. There is an area of calcification overlying the cardiac silhouette (arrowed). This represents a calcified aortic valve, although it is impossible to say this with certainty without doing a lateral view.
The lung fields contain a generalised increase in vascular markings, and in particular the upper lobe blood vessels look bulky.
Soft tissues — normal
Pleura and diaphragm — normal.
Bony structures — normal.
Conclusion. Calcific aortic stenosis, with secondary increase in pulmonary venous pressure.

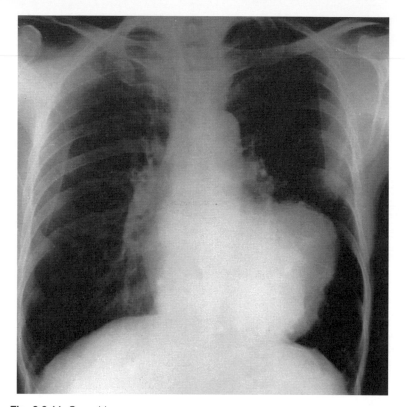

Fig. 3.2.11 Case 11.

This is a PA chest radiograph.

Cardiothoracic ratio = 0.56 (abnormal).

There is cardiomegaly. The main area of cardiac enlargement is on the left side of the cardiac outline, which also appears to have a double shadow. The left border of the heart is considerably 'bowed-out' (convex outwards).

Lung fields — normal.

Soft tissues — normal.

Pleura and diaphragm — normal.

Bony structures — normal.

Conclusion. Left ventricular enlargement due to a cardiac aneurysm.

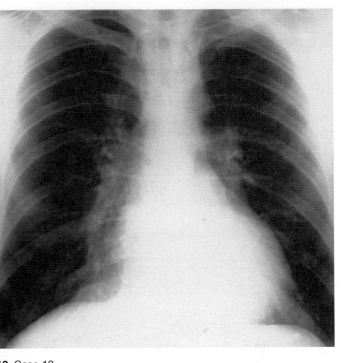

Fig. 3.2.12 Case 12.

This is a PA chest radiograph.
Mediastinum — normal.
Lung fields — normal.
Soft tissues — normal.
Pleura and diaphragm — normal.
Bony structures — abnormal.
Conclusion. This radiograph demonstrates classical rib
notching, as found in coarctation of the aorta. This is seen on
the inferior surfaces of the ribs, overlying the mid-zones of
both lung fields.

This radiograph does not demonstrate the other radiological
feature of coarctation — post-stenotic dilatation of the aorta.
This would be seen as an enlargement of the mediastinal
shadow in the area between the aortic knuckle and the left
hilum. This case illustrates the necessity of looking carefully
and methodically at all areas of the radiograph.

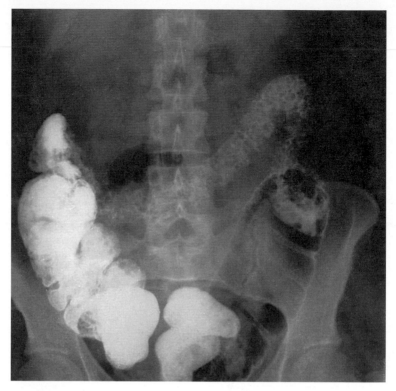

Fig. 3.2.13 Case 13.

This is a barium enema examination.

The transverse colon shows a grossly abnormal appearance. Throughout the whole of the transverse and proximal descending colon there is severe and continuous mucosal ulceration and oedema. There is loss of the normal haustral pattern in this region. The abnormalities show sparing of the ascending colon.

Conclusion. These findings are in keeping with the diagnosis of ulcerative colitis.

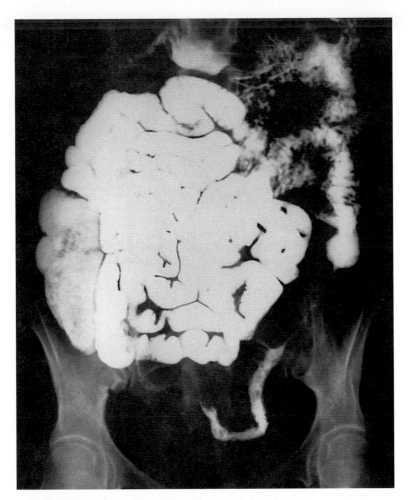

Fig. 3.2.14 Case 14.

This is a small bowel contrast study.

Barium outlines the small bowel. In addition there is a small amount of contrast in the stomach and duodenal cap (top of the picture).

There is an area of stricturing of the small bowel (overlying the left sacroiliac joint). Proximal to this there is a short length of bowel with abnormal mucosa. This demonstrates mucosal oedema and ulceration, including several 'rose-thorn' ulcers.

Conclusion. These findings are compatible with Crohn's disease.

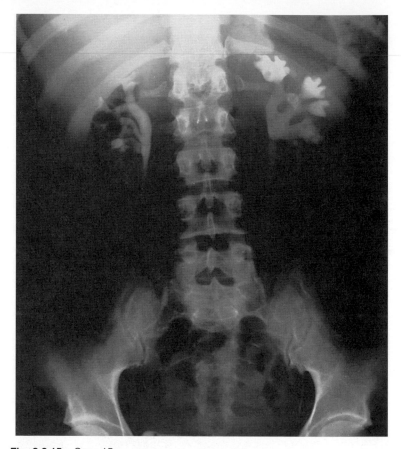

Fig. 3.2.15a Case 15a.

This is an intravenous urogram (IVU).

Contrast is seen in both pelvicalyceal systems and proximal ureters.

The left ureter can just be seen in the pelvis.

The left pelvicalyceal system is slightly dilated, compared with the right.

Bladder — not seen.

Bony structures — normal.

Soft tissues — normal.

Conclusion. Slight enlargement of the left pelvicalyceal system, cause unknown.

If you are asked to comment on an IVU, always ask to see a control film (a plain radiograph, before contrast was given). Please see Case 15b.

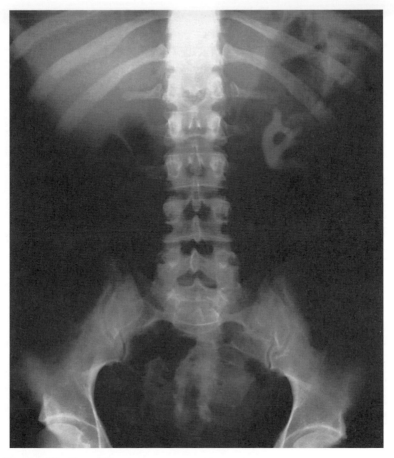

Fig. 3.2.15b Case 15b.

This is a control film for the IVU shown in Case 15a, and was therefore taken before the injection of contrast. The cause of the minimal dilatation of the left pelvicalyceal system is now obvious. There is a large staghorn calculus on the left.
Note. It is impossible to make this diagnosis from the IVU alone, without seeing the control film.

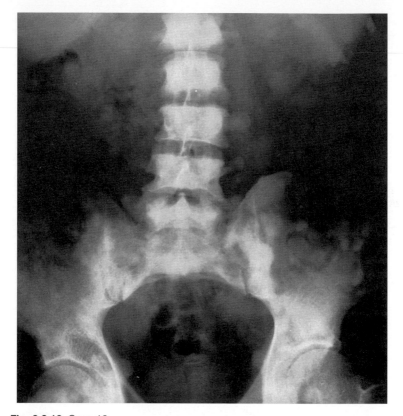

Fig. 3.2.16 Case 16.

This is a plain radiograph of the pelvis.
There are sclerotic deposits throughout the lumbar spine and pelvis.
Conclusion. This appearance is seen in carcinoma of:

- prostate
- breast
- thyroid.

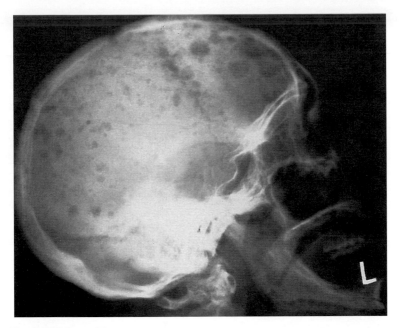

Fig. 3.2.17 Case 17.

This is a lateral skull radiograph.
There are multiple circular defects of varying sizes throughout the vault of the skull. These also affect the mandible.
Conclusion. This is a characteristic appearance of multiple myeloma.

Note. Causes of 'holes' in the vault of the skull include:

- congenital
- malignant tumours
  — myeloma
  — metastatic carcinoma
  — lymphoma
- benign tumours
  — neurofibroma
- arteriovenous malformations.

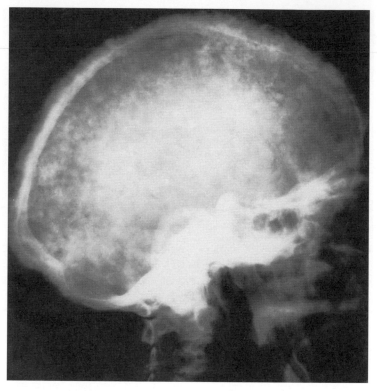

Fig. 3.2.18 Case 18.

This is a lateral skull radiograph.
There are multiple, fluffy opacities throughout the skull.
Conclusion. This 'cotton wool' effect is characteristic of
Paget's disease.

3.3

Certifying death

Certifying death is a core clinical skill which you may need from day 1 as a doctor. To certify a patient dead, the following are required:

- patient unresponsive
- absence of carotid pulse over 1 minute
- absence of breath sounds over 1 minute
- pupils dilated and unreactive to light.

Note. Use of adrenaline at a cardiac arrest can cause dilated pupils and this needs to be borne in mind when certifying death in this situation.

When you have completed your examination, remember to leave your patient (usually a mannequin) in a dignified manner. This means covering the body up to the neck with a sheet or blanket. Always record the date and time of death in the notes, and make arrangements for relatives to be informed.

Certification of brain stem death is a more complex procedure and it is unlikely that you will be asked to do this at an OSCE; however, students have been asked about it in the past. Tests used to certify brain stem death include:

- pupil reaction
- corneal reflex
- eye movements on caloric testing
- gag reflex
- cough reflex
- respiratory effort when taken off the ventilator.

These tests must be performed by two independent experienced doctors (at least 5 years post-registration), one of whom must be a consultant.

The timing of brain stem death tests is as follows:

- at least 1 hour apart
- >6 hours after onset of coma
- >24 hours post-cardiac arrest.

WRITING A DEATH CERTIFICATE

This is a common question. Remember the following tips:

- Always write in block capitals.
- Write the patient's full name.
- When writing the date of death, put the date in words.
- Write cause rather than mode of death (coma, syncope, cardiac arrest, etc. are modes of death).
- Remember to check the patient's employment history, as some industrial diseases attract financial compensation.
- If you do not know the cause of death, you may not be able to issue a death certificate.

Some patients need to be referred to the coroner. Reasons for referring to the coroner include:

- cause of death unknown
- patient not seen by the certifying doctor either after death or within 14 days before death
- death was violent/unnatural/suspicious
- accidental deaths
- suicide
- neglect/self-neglect
- industrial disease
- death in prison/custody
- death during an operation.

We have included several examples for you to consider. The answers can be found on the following page.

Case 1

Mrs Gillian Roper is an 88-year-old woman with a medical history of hypertension and rheumatoid arthritis. She has a history of transient ischaemic attacks for which she takes 75 mg of aspirin in addition to 5 mg of lisinopril for hypertension. Her rheumatoid arthritis is burnt out and she is on no medication for this.

She was admitted 5 days ago with a dense left hemiparesis. A CT scan showed a right middle cerebral artery infarction with oedema.

She was treated actively but, despite this, her level of consciousness deteriorated and on full discussion with the family she was kept comfortable and died on 14 May 2001. You were the house physician looking after her who certified her at death.

MOCK MEDICAL CERTIFICATE OF CAUSE OF DEATH

Name of deceased. GILLIAN ROPER

Date of death. FOURTEENTH ....day of.. MAY 2001 .....Age. 80

Place of death. SAINT SWITHINS HOSPITAL, LONDON

Last seen alive by me. FOURTEENTH ....day of MAY 2001

1   The certified cause of death takes account
    of information obtained from post-mortem

2   Information from post mortem
    may be available later

3   Post-mortem not being held

4   I have reported this death to the coroner
    for further action

please ring
appropriate
digits
and letters

a   Seen after death by me
b   Seen after death by another medical practitioner
c   Not seen after death by a medical practitioner

CAUSE OF DEATH

I (a) Disease or condition directly CEREBROVASCULAR EVENT (STROKE)
     leading to death.

(b) Other disease or condition, if any, leading to I (a). HYPERTENSION

(c) Other disease or condition, if any, leading to I (b).

II Other significant conditions
    contributing but not related   RHEUMATOID ARTHRITIS
    to the disease causing it.

The death might have been due to or contributed to by the employment followed at some time by the deceased

Please tick if applicable

Signature. DSWatson   D. S. WATSON   Date. 15/5/01

Fig. 3.3.1 Case 1.

Case 2

Mr Michael Hunt is a 76-year-old retired farmer who has smoked all his life. He was diagnosed with maturity onset diabetes mellitus 10 years ago, for which he takes maximal doses of oral hypoglycaemics. He was admitted on one occasion to convert him to insulin but could not manage this and refused district nurse assistance.

For the last 5 years he has had ischaemic heart disease, getting angina on moderate exertion. He has been admitted twice in the last year with cardiac chest pain and had a positive exercise treadmill test after 4 minutes of standard Bruce protocol. He declined angiography and would not entertain the idea of coronary bypass grafting.

He was admitted 2 days ago with a massive anterolateral myocardial infarction for which he received thrombolysis. Despite this, he went into cardiogenic shock and died despite full inotropic support.

He died at 7 o'clock in the morning on 7 May 2001. Your SHO pronounced him dead.

MOCK MEDICAL CERTIFICATE OF CAUSE OF DEATH

Name of deceased... MICHAEL HUNT

Date of death... SEVENTH ...day of... MAY 2001 ...Age... 76

Place of death... ST SWITHINS HOSPITAL, LONDON

Last seen alive by me... SIXTH ...day of... MAY 2001

1 The certified cause of death takes account
 of information obtained from post-mortem

2 Information from post mortem
 may be available later
 Post-mortem not being held

4 I have reported this death to the coroner
 for further action

{   please ring
    appropriate
    digits
    and letters

{   a   Seen after death by me
    b   Seen after death by another medical practitioner
    c   Not seen after death by a medical practitioner

CAUSE OF DEATH

I (a) Disease or condition directly
 leading to death... MYOCARDIAL INFARCTION

(b) Other disease or condition, if any, leading to I (a) ... ISCHAEMIC HEART DISEASE

(c) Other disease or condition, if any, leading to I (b) ... DIABETES MELLITUS

II Other significant conditions
 contributing but not related
 to the disease causing it.

The death might have been due to or contributed to by the employment followed at some time by the deceased.

Please tick if applicable ☐

Signature... DS Watson O.S. WATSON ...Date... 7/5/01

Fig. 3.3.2 Case 2.

Case 3

Mr Thomas Foley is a 39-year-old librarian who presented 2 weeks ago with an atypical chest infection and ataxia. He was subsequently diagnosed as having *Pneumocystis carinii* pneumonia and a viral encephalitis of unknown origin. He was found to be human immunodeficiency virus antibody-positive with a CD4 count of 8 and a very high viral load.

He was treated with triple therapy, Septrin and aciclovir.

During his stay he had a grand mal seizure and subsequent cardiac arrest. In accordance with his living will and requests on admission, he was not subjected to prolonged cardiopulmonary resuscitation or ventilation. His parents were unaware of his diagnosis. You pronounced him dead at 16.40 hours on 6 July 2001.

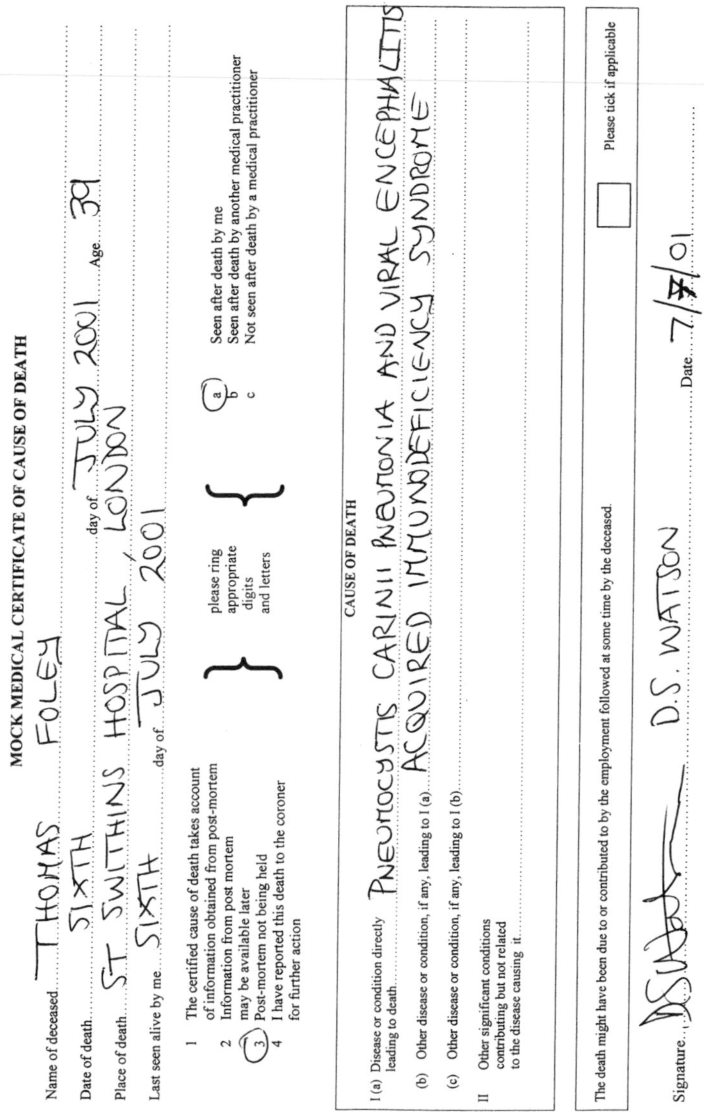

MOCK MEDICAL CERTIFICATE OF CAUSE OF DEATH

Name of deceased ...... THOMAS FOLEY

Date of death ...... SIXTH ...... day of ...... JULY 2001 ...... Age ... 39

Place of death ...... ST SWITHINS HOSPITAL, LONDON

Last seen alive by me ...... SIXTH ...... day of ...... JULY 2001

1 The certified cause of death takes account
of information obtained from post-mortem
2 Information from post mortem
may be available later
③ Post-mortem not being held
4 I have reported this death to the coroner
for further action

please ring
appropriate
digits
and letters

ⓐ Seen after death by me
b Seen after death by another medical practitioner
c Not seen after death by a medical practitioner

CAUSE OF DEATH

I (a) Disease or condition directly ... PNEUMOCYSTIS CARINII PNEUMONIA AND VIRAL ENCEPHALITIS
leading to death

(b) Other disease or condition, if any, leading to I (a) ... ACQUIRED IMMUNODEFICIENCY SYNDROME

(c) Other disease or condition, if any, leading to I (b) ......

II Other significant conditions
contributing but not related
to the disease causing it. ......

The death might have been due to or contributed to by the employment followed at some time by the deceased.

Please tick if applicable ☐

Signature ...... D.S. WATSON ...... Date ... 7/7/01

Fig. 3.3.3 Case 3.

Case 4

Mr Arthur Jessup is a 72-year-old man who has been seen yearly for follow-up in the respiratory clinic for asbestos-related pulmonary fibrosis. This was thought to be due to time he spent as a dock worker in the 1940s.

He had a past medical history of cholecystectomy and right inguinal hernia repair. He was due to have his left hernia repaired but was thought to be too great an anaesthetic risk.

He had his follow-up appointment expedited as he had become increasingly short of breath and was getting pain on inspiration. He was admitted directly from clinic to the ward where he was found to have a large right-sided pleural effusion with extensive pleural calcification which had changed significantly from the previous films.

Pleural aspiration and biopsy revealed an abundance of malignant cells consistent with mesothelioma.

He deteriorated quickly during his in-patient stay, receiving one dose of palliative radiotherapy to help with chest pain. Date of death as certified by you was 21 May 2001.

MOCK MEDICAL CERTIFICATE OF CAUSE OF DEATH

Name of deceased ..... ARTHUR JESSUP .....

Date of death ..... TWENTY FIRST ..... day of ..... MAY 2001 ..... Age ..... 72 .....

Place of death ..... ST. SWITHINS HOSPITAL LONDON .....

Last seen alive by me ..... TWENTY FIRST ..... day of ..... MAY 2001 .....

1 The certified cause of death takes account
of information obtained from post-mortem

2 Information from post mortem
may be available later

3 Post-mortem not being held

4 I have reported this death to the coroner
for further action

please ring
appropriate
digits
and letters

(a) Seen after death by me
b   Seen after death by another medical practitioner
c   Not seen after death by a medical practitioner

CAUSE OF DEATH

I (a) Disease or condition directly
leading to death ..... MESOTHELIOMA .....

(b) Other disease or condition, if any, leading to I (a) ..... ASBESTOSIS .....

(c) Other disease or condition, if any, leading to I (b) .....

II   Other significant conditions
contributing but not related
to the disease causing it .....

The death might have been due to or contributed to by the employment followed at some time by the deceased.   ☑ Please tick if applicable

Signature ..... D.S. WATSON .....   Date ..... 22/5/00 .....

Fig. 3.3.4 Case 4.

Case 5

Mr Syed Sumendra is a 70-year-old Muslim who was admitted on 28 July 2001 at 8 p.m. He presented to the accident and emergency department with severe central chest pain and pain in the upper abdomen. He had a past history of diabetes mellitus and hypertension for which he took gliclazide 80 mg b.d., frusemide 40 mg o.d., and lisinopril 5 mg o.d. Prior to admission his wife told you that he had symptoms which were suggestive of intermittent claudication in the right calf.

Clinical examination showed the patient to be in extreme pain, sweaty, tachycardic, with a blood pressure of 80/40. There was generalised abdominal tenderness in the upper abdomen but bowel sounds were normal.

Initial investigation showed him to have a normal chest X-ray and a normal abdominal X-ray; full blood count revealed a haemoglobin of 10, white count of 5, platelet count of 460.

You strongly suspected that this patient had a ruptured abdominal aortic aneurysm and immediately called the surgical registrar. However, before the surgical registrar could see the patient, he had a cardiac arrest from which he could not be resuscitated.

After pronouncing death and recording it in the notes, you see the relatives to break the bad news. The family are very keen for an early burial and would like you to write a death certificate.

You cannot issue a death certificate on this patient, as you do not know the cause of death. You must refer this case to the coroner.

CREMATION FORMS

The principles of completing a cremation form are similar to those of completing a death certificate. However, you must remember the following:

- You must see the body after death.
- You must be certain that the patient has not died through violence, privation or neglect.
- You must ensure that the patient does not have:
  — a pacemaker   } These need to be removed prior to
  — a radioactive implant } cremation.

In essence you are signing a legal document which states that it is safe to cremate the body and that it will not need to be exhumed in 10 years' time. We recommend you get hold of some specimen cremation certificates and fill them in, prior to taking your examination.

Interpreting blood test results

Interpreting blood test results is an increasingly commonly asked practical OSCE question in Final MB. It is an important skill to have, as you will need to be able to do this from day 1 of your professional life. The questions are usually given as a brief scenario.

We have included a number of questions together with answers and explanations.

Question 1

A 45-year-old man attends his family doctor complaining of feeling tired all the time and of muscle weakness. His blood test results are as follows:

Na	126 mmol/l	(135–145 mmol/l)
K	6.1 mmol/l	(3.5–5.0 mmol/l)
Urea	9.6 mmol/l	(2.5–8.0 mmol/l)
Creatinine	150 µmol/l	(40–130 µmol/l)

How would you explain these blood test results?

Answer

This patient has a low sodium, high potassium and mild renal impairment. The common causes of this blood picture are:

- potassium-sparing diuretic
- mineralocorticoid deficiency, e.g. Addison's disease.

The way to make an accurate diagnosis is to take a complete drug history and to perform a short Synacthen test, if the patient is not taking a potassium-sparing diuretic.

Common causes of hyperkalaemia

- Haemolysis[a]
- Potassium-sparing diuretic
- Addison's disease
- Renal failure
- Metabolic acidosis.

[a]This is the commonest cause of hyperkalaemia in clinical practice. It is caused by red cell lysis in a blood sample that has been left too long before processing by the laboratory. As the red cells lyse, they leak potassium into the serum, producing an erroneously high result. Most laboratories will report whether the sample was haemolysed and recommend repeat sampling.

Common causes of hyponatraemia

See Question 4, page 230.

Question 2

A 40-year-old man has a blood pressure of 165/105. His blood test results are as follows:

Na	142 mmol/l	(135–145 mmol/l)
K	3.0 mmol/l	(3.5–5.0 mmol/l)
HCO₃	30 mmol/l	(21–28 mmol/l)
Cl	104 mmol/l	(95–105 mmol/l)
Urea	6.4 mmol/l	(2.5–8.0 mmol/l)
Creatinine	110 µmol/l	(40–130 µmol/l)

How would you explain these blood test results?

Answer

This patient has a low potassium and a raised bicarbonate (hypokalaemic alkalosis).

Causes of a hypokalaemic alkalosis

- Conn's syndrome
- Bilateral renal artery stenosis
- Diuretic therapy
- Corticosteroid therapy
- Cushing's syndrome
- Persistent vomiting

- Purgative abuse
- Liquorice ingestion.

As the patient is hypertensive the most likely cause in this patient is one of the first five causes in the above list.

Conn's syndrome, or primary hyperaldosteronism, is caused by excessive secretion of aldosterone, usually from an adenoma in the adrenal gland. It is a very rare cause of secondary hypertension.

Bilateral renal artery stenosis is another uncommon cause of secondary hypertension. It causes hypertension by causing hyperaldosteronism because of reduced renal perfusion, which stimulates the renal–angiotensin system.

Diuretic therapy is not a cause of hypertension, but over 50% of patients with this condition take diuretic therapy to treat their high blood pressure. It is possible that this patient is already being treated for his hypertension. Diuretic therapy is the most likely explanation for his blood test results.

Excessive corticosteroids, either iatrogenic or due to Cushing's disease, are another cause of (usually mild) hypertension and hypokalaemia.

Question 3

A 56-year-old alcoholic is admitted to hospital with a collapse. He is inebriated and unable to give a history. His blood test results are as follows:

Na	135 mmol/l	(135–145 mmol/l)
K	3.6 mmol/l	(3.5–5.0 mmol/l)
Urea	16.0 mmol/l	(2.5–8.0 mmol/l)
Creatinine	62 µmol/l	(40–130 µmol/l)

How would you explain these blood test results?

Answer

This patient has a high urea, but a normal creatinine (raised urea/creatinine ratio).

Causes of a raised urea:creatinine ratio

- Upper gastrointestinal bleed
- Dehydration

- Corticosteroid therapy
- Tetracycline therapy.

In an alcoholic with this blood picture the diagnosis is an upper gastrointestinal bleed until proven otherwise. The gut digests the large volume of blood in the gastrointestinal tract. The increase in the urea: creatinine ratio in this situation is due to the large protein load in the upper gastrointestinal tract.

It is essential to do a rectal examination in this patient, as there may be melaena stool on the examining glove. It is also important to check his full blood count as he may have evidence of anaemia secondary to the gastrointestinal bleed.

Question 4

An 86-year-old woman is admitted to hospital with a fractured neck of femur. Two days post-operatively she becomes increasingly confused. Her blood test results are as follows:

Na	116 mmol/l	(135–145 mmol/l)
K	3.8 mmol/l	(3.5–5.0 mmol/l)
Urea	4.6 mmol/l	(2.5–8.0 mmol/l)
Creatinine	92 μmol/l	(40–130 μmol/l)

How would you explain these blood test results?

Answer

This patient has a very low sodium. Hyponatraemia at this kind of level can cause quite profound confusion, particularly in the elderly.

Causes of hyponatraemia

- Sodium loss
  — vomiting
  — diarrhoea
  — enteric fistula
  — Addison's disease
  — drugs, e.g. diuretics
- Water retention
  — inappropriate choice of intravenous fluids
  — nephrotic syndrome

- congestive cardiac failure
- syndrome of inappropriate antidiuretic hormone secretion (SIADH)
- compulsive water drinking.

The most likely cause in this patient is inappropriate intravenous fluid replacement in the perioperative period. This is particularly common in patients who are given 5% dextrose or dextrose/saline.

In an elderly patient with hyponatraemia, inappropriate antidiuretic hormone secretion (SIADH) should always be considered because several of the causes are commonly found in the elderly population.

Causes of inappropriate antidiuretic hormone secretion (SIADH)

- Abscess
  - lung
  - brain
  - abdominal
- Infection
  - respiratory
  - meningitis
- Pulmonary tuberculosis
- Stroke
- Lung cancer
- Head injury
- Drugs
  - sulphonamides
  - SSRIs
  - omeprazole.

The diagnosis of SIADH is confirmed by measuring the osmolality in paired serum and urine samples. In patients with SIADH the osmolality of the serum is low, and the osmolality of the urine is inappropriately high for the serum osmolality. The mechanism for this is excessive water retention by the kidneys driven by inappropriately high levels of antidiuretic hormone in the serum.

Question 5

An 18-year-old girl collapses at school. Her blood test results are as follows:

Na	135 mmol/l	(135–145 mmol/l)
K	3.2 mmol/l	(3.5–5.0 mmol/l)
Urea	1.9 mmol/l	(2.5–8.0 mmol/l)
Creatinine	37 μmol/l	(40–130 μmol/l)

How would you explain these blood test results?

Answer

This patient has a low urea and creatinine. In a patient with normal renal function the urea and creatinine are a reflection of protein intake and muscle bulk.

Causes of a low urea and creatinine

- Anorexia nervosa
- Disseminated cancer
- Alcohol dependence syndrome (poor diet)
- Protein-calorie malnutrition
- Severe malabsorption.

This patient needs a full medical assessment to determine the cause of her collapse and the blood picture. Although anorexia nervosa is the most likely diagnosis, other causes need to be excluded first.

Question 6

A 26-year-old man goes to see his doctor complaining of 'yellow jaundice'. His blood test results are as follows:

ALKP	262 U/l	(30–105 U/l)
ALT	4526 U/l	(15–35 U/l)
Bilirubin	196 μmol/l	(3–17 μmol/l)

How would you explain these blood test results?

Answer

This patient has a very elevated ALT and bilirubin and a modestly elevated ALKP. When the ALT is elevated out of proportion to the ALKP, as in this case, this suggests an acute hepatocellular cause for the jaundice.

Common causes of acute hepatocellular jaundice in a 26-year-old man

- Acute viral hepatitis
  - — acute hepatitis A
  - — acute hepatitis B
- Drug-induced liver injury
  - — recreational — ecstasy
  - — iatrogenic — e.g. antibiotics, NSAIDs
  - — overdose — paracetamol
- Acute alcoholic hepatitis (ALT is often not very high in this condition).

Question 7

A 76-year-old man goes to see his doctor complaining of 'yellow jaundice'. His blood test results are as follows:

ALKP	1262 U/l	(30–105 U/l)
ALT	262 U/l	(15–35 U/l)
Bilirubin	196 µmol/l	(3–17 µmol/l)

How would you explain these blood test results?

Answer

This patient has a very elevated ALKP and bilirubin and a modestly elevated ALT. When the ALKP is elevated out of proportion to the ALT, as in this case, this suggests a cholestatic cause for the jaundice. This cholestatic picture is caused by biliary obstruction. The obstruction is either post-hepatic (bile duct level) or at the level of the biliary canaliculi (cholestatic hepatocellular jaundice). In the former the biliary tree is dilated on transabdominal ultrasound, and in the latter it is not.

Common causes of acute cholestatic jaundice in a 76-year-old man

- Biliary obstruction (dilated bile ducts on ultrasound)
  - — carcinoma of the head of the pancreas
  - — common bile duct stone
- Cholestatic hepatocellular jaundice (non-dilated bile ducts on ultrasound)
  - — drug reaction e.g. flucloxacillin, co-amoxiclav[a]

— metastatic disease

— primary sclerosing cholangitis.

[a]Drug-induced cholestatic hepatocellular injury is common with these antibiotics. Elderly (>65 years) male patients are particularly prone to drug-induced jaundice after treatment with flucloxacillin or co-amoxiclav. These antibiotics should be used with caution in this group of patients.

Question 8

A 65-year-old woman has been feeling progressively unwell for several weeks. Her blood test results are as follows:

ALKP	242 U/l	(30–105 U/l)
Corrected calcium	3.52 mmol/l	(2.2–2.6 mmol/l)
PO$_4$	1.0 mmol/l	(0.7–1.4 mmol/l)

How would you explain these blood test results?

Answer

This patient has a very high serum corrected calcium and a high ALKP. The phosphate is normal.

Causes of hypercalcaemia

- Primary hyperparathyroidism
- Malignancy
- Myeloma
- Sarcoidosis
- Vitamin D excess
- Thyrotoxicosis (rare).

Hypercalcaemia associated with malignancy is the commonest cause of a raised calcium in a hospital population. It is most commonly caused by secretion of parathyroid hormone-related protein. This causes an increase in bone turnover due to upregulation of osteoclastic activity and hence hypercalcaemia. Although commonly associated with bony metastases, several potentially resectable primary tumours, such as squamous cell carcinoma of the lung, also secrete it. Therefore, in a patient with hypercalcaemia due to lung cancer, the hypercalcaemia does not necessarily imply incurable disease.

Question 9

A 45-year-old woman goes to see her doctor with weight gain. Her blood test results are as follows:

TSH	95 mU/l	(0.5–5.0 mU/l)
T_4	23 nmol/l	(55–144 nmol/l)

How would you explain these blood test results?

Answer

This patient has a very high serum TSH and a low T_4. This is compatible with a diagnosis of hypothyroidism. Hypothyroidism is a relatively common cause of weight gain in a woman of this age, although overeating and lack of exercise are the usual culprits.

Causes of hypothyroidism

- Autoimmune
- Following treatment for hyperthyroidism
  - partial thyroidectomy
  - radioiodine therapy
- Drugs, e.g. lithium, amiodarone
- Severe iodine deficiency.

Question 10

A 24-year-old woman presents with acute shortness of breath. Her blood gas results are as follows:

pH	7.52	(7.35–7.45)
PCO_2	2.9 kPa	(4.4–5.6 kPa)
PO_2	13.6 kPa	(12–15 kPa)
HCO_3	31 mmol/l	(21–28 mmol/l)

How would you explain these results?

Answer

This patient has a respiratory alkalosis with a raised pH and HCO_3, a low PCO_2 and a normal PO_2. The most likely explanation is that she has been hyperventilating. A rapid respiratory rate will lead her to blow off her PCO_2. This results in a hypocapnic alkalosis.

Question 11

A 24-year-old woman presents with acute shortness of breath and pleuritic chest pain. Her blood gas results are as follows:

pH	7.52	(7.35–7.45)
P_{CO_2}	2.9 kPa	(4.4–5.6 kPa)
P_{O_2}	9.1 kPa	(12–15 kPa)
HCO_3	28 mmol/l	(21–28 mmol/l)

How would you explain these results?

Answer

These results are very similar to the previous question except that the patient is hypoxic. It is likely that the hypoxia has caused the patient to hyperventilate, causing a secondary reduction in P_{CO_2} and a rise in pH.

This patient, therefore, has acute dyspnoea, pleuritic chest pain and hypoxia. The cause of this is a pulmonary embolism until proven otherwise.

Question 12

A 60-year-old smoker presents with gradually increasing shortness of breath. His blood gas results are as follows:

pH	7.35	(7.35–7.45)
P_{CO_2}	9.0 kPa	(4.4–5.6 kPa)
P_{O_2}	5.0 kPa	(12–15 kPa)
HCO_3	40 mmol/l	(21–28 mmol/l)

How would you explain these results?

Answer

This patient has a high P_{CO_2} and a low P_{O_2} suggesting hypoventilation. This has led to a respiratory acidosis because of the build-up of CO_2. However, the pH is normal and the HCO_3 is raised, indicating metabolic compensation (bicarbonate preserved by the kidneys to offset the respiratory acidosis).

This is type II respiratory failure and is usually caused by chronic obstructive pulmonary disease. Oxygen therapy must be used with caution in this kind of patient. Hypoxia is driving the patient's respiratory efforts. Treating a patient like this with oxygen at high concentrations can take away the hypoxic drive, resulting in cardio-respiratory collapse.

Question 13

A 24-year-old woman is admitted to hospital with general malaise, weight loss and thirst. Her blood gas results are as follows:

pH	7.12	(7.35–7.45)
P_{CO_2}	2.6 kPa	(4.4–5.6 kPa)
P_{O_2}	13.6 kPa	(12–15 kPa)
HCO_3	8 mmol/l	(21–28 mmol/l)

How would you explain these results?

Answer

This patient has a low pH, HCO_3 and P_{CO_2} with a normal P_{O_2}. This is a metabolic acidosis. The P_{CO_2} is low due to a secondary increased respiratory drive in an attempt to compensate for the metabolic acidosis. This patient is very sick. You need to seek advice from a senior colleague.

Causes of a metabolic acidosis

- Diabetic ketoacidosis
- Lactic acidosis, including sepsis
- Renal disease
- Poisoning
  - — methanol
  - — salicylate.

KEY QUESTIONS

Interpreting blood test results

We have included a number of other questions for you to consider which you may encounter in the Final MB examination. If you have difficulty with any of the answers (and one or two of them are quite tricky and are marked with an asterisk) you can always look up the answers in a reference text. Failing that, the answers can be found in *Best of Five for MRCP*, Fellows HJ, Noble SIR and Dalton HR, Elsevier. The question number in parentheses refers to the question and answer number as they appear in the first edition (2005) of this book.

1 (11). **A 51-year-old patient with rheumatoid arthritis is admitted with pneumococcal pneumonia.** On examination she has splenomegaly and the following blood test results:

Hb	10 g/dl	(12–16 g/dl)
WCC	2.1×10^9/l	($4–11 \times 10^9$/l)
Platelets	123×10^9/l	($150–400 \times 10^9$/l)

What is the most likely diagnosis?

2 (21). **These were the test results from blood taken at a routine clinic attendance:**

Na	138 mmol/l	(135–145 mmol/l)
K	4.0 mmol/l	(3.5–5.0 mmol/l)
Cl	108 mmol/l	(95–106 mmol/l)
Bicarbonate	20 mmol/l	(22–30 mmol/l)
Urea	6.8 mmol/l	(2.5–6.7 mmol/l)
Creatinine	108 µmol/l	(70–150 µmol/l)

What is the correct value of the anion gap?

3* (31). **A 67-year-old man presents with nausea and pain in his right upper quadrant.** On examination he has tender hepatomegaly with an irregular edge. His blood test results are as follows.

Hb 8 g/dl	(11.5–16 g/dl)
WCC 17.8×10^9/l	($4–11 \times 10^9$/l)
Platelets 104×10^9/l	($150–400 \times 10^9$/l)
Neutrophils 68%	

Normoblasts 8%
Myeloblasts 8%
Myelocytes 5%
Metamyelocytes 5%
Lymphocytes 15%

How would you explain these results?

4 (44). A 19-year-old woman presents with severe tiredness. Three weeks ago she had a serious chest infection that was treated with a full course of antibiotics. Her blood test results are:

Hb	9.3 g/dl	(12–16 g/dl)
MCV	98 fl	(85–96 fl)
MCH	28 g/dl	(32–35 g/dl)
WBC	7.8×10^9/l	$(4–11 \times 10^9$/l)
Platelets	178×10^9/l	$(150–400 \times 10^9$/l)
Reticulocytes	9%	(<1%)
Monospot	Negative	
Blood film	Polychromasia, autoagglutination Microspherocytes	

How would you explain these results?

5 (275). A 38-year-old nurse is referred with symptoms of tiredness, nausea and a change in weight. Her thyroid function tests are as follows:

T_3	3.4 nmol/l	(0.9–2.8 nmol/l)
T_4	177 nmol/l	(55–144 nmol/l)
TSH	1.2 mU/l	(0.35–5.0 mU/l)
TBG	37 mg/l	(12–30 mg/l)

How would you explain these results?

6 (304). A 74-year-old man presents to an orthopaedic pre-clerking clinic while awaiting his total hip replacement. He is otherwise fit and well. Examination is unremarkable. His blood test results are as follows:

Hb	17.2 g/dl	(13–18 g/dl)
WCC	29×10^9/l	$(4–11 \times 10^9$/l)
Platelets	180×10^9/l	$(150–400 \times 10^9$/l)
MCV	90 fl	(76–96 fl)

Differential:

Lymphocytes $16.4 \times 10^9/l$ $(1.3–3.5 \times 10^9/l)$

Neutrophils $6.5 \times 10^9/l$ $(2–7.5 \times 10^9/l)$

How would you explain these results?

7 (272). **A 76-year-old man presents to his GP with weight loss and anorexia.** Examination reveals splenomegaly. Blood test results are as follows:

Hb	10.8 g/dl	(13–18 g/dl)
WCC	$95.9 \times 10^9/l$	$(4–11 \times 10^9/l)$
Platelets	$125 \times 10^9/l$	$(150–400 \times 10^9/l)$
Blood film	Myelocytes, metamyelocytes and myeloblasts	

How would you explain these results?

8 (227). **A 6-year-old child is investigated for easy bruising.** Blood test results are as follows:

Prothrombin time	13 s	(12–15.5 s)
APTT	86 s	(30–46 s)
Thrombin time	12 s	(15–19 s)
Bleeding time	6 min	(2–8 min)

What is the most likely diagnosis?

9* (192). **A 45-year-old man with anaemia is referred to a gastroenterologist by his GP.** The patient is asymptomatic and his blood test results are as follows:

Hb	9.6 g/dl	(13–18 g/dl)
WCC	$4.2 \times 10^9/l$	$(4–11 \times 10^9/l)$
Platelets	$158 \times 10^9/l$	$(150–400 \times 10^9/l)$
MCV	60 fl	(76–96 fl)
Ferritin	35 µg/l	(12–200 µg/l)
Blood film	Hypochromic, microcytic	

Which investigation should be performed next?

10* (136). **A 55-year-old man presents to his GP with a 2-month history of tiredness and lethargy.** Initial blood tests are as follows:

Hb	9.2 g/dl	(13–18 g/dl)
WCC	$7.1 \times 10^9/l$	$(4–11 \times 10^9/l)$
Platelets	$243 \times 10^9/l$	$(150–400 \times 10^9/l)$

MCV	96 fl	(76–96 fl)
Total protein	78 g/l	(60–80 g/l)
Albumin	30 g/l	(35–50 g/l)
Na	133 mmol/l	(135–145 mmol/l)
K	5.5 mmol/l	(3.5–5 mmol/l)
Urea	16.4 mmol/l	(2.5–6.7 mmol/l)
Creatinine	254 μmol/l	(70–150 μmol/l)

What is the most likely diagnosis?

11 (54). **A 50-year-old woman presents with tiredness.** Full blood count and film results are:

Hb	8.2 g/dl	(12–16 g/dl)
WCC	5.2×10^9/l	$(4–11 \times 10^9$/l)
Platelets	342×10^9/l	$(150–400 \times 10^9$/l)
Blood film	Macrocytes and microcytes seen	
	Target cells and Howell–Jolly bodies	
	Irregularly contracted red cells	

What is the most likely diagnosis?

12* (338). **Which drug is most likely to result in the blood test results shown below?**

Na	141 mmol/l	(135–145 mmol/l)
K	3.3 mmol/l	(3.5–5.0 mmol/l)
Cl	118 mmol/l	(95–106 mmol/l)
HCO_3	13 mmol/l	(22–30 mmol/l)
Urea	6.8 mmol/l	(2.5–6.7 mmol/l)
Creatinine	108 μmol/l	(70–150 μmol/l)

3.5

Other practical OSCE stations

There is a large range of practical OSCE stations which you could potentially meet. We address the more commonly asked questions in the following pages. Remember that when doing any OSCE which involves patient contact, marks will be awarded for conduct, professionalism and communication skills in addition to the procedure itself. In some medical schools, discretionary marks are also awarded for 'overall performance'.

BASIC LIFE SUPPORT ☠

This is an essential skill which is commonly tested and could well be a death station. It is a skill that is best learned by practising repeatedly so that it becomes second nature. We strongly recommend that you approach your hospital's resuscitation training officer and ensure that you are taken through basic life support according to the UK resuscitation guidelines. What follows is by no means a comprehensive guide to basic life support but will hopefully serve as an *aide-mémoire* for the basic approach with which you can practise and develop your skills.

Sequence of actions = A B C

- Ensure it is safe to approach.
- Check the patient and see if there is a response — if the patient does not respond, shout for assistance.
- Airway — open the **A**irway by head tilt and chin lift.
- Keeping the airway open, look, listen and feel for **B**reathing for 10 seconds.
- If the patient is breathing, place in the recovery position; if the patient is not breathing, go for help. The most treatable cause of cardiac arrest is ventricular fibrillation, which requires immediate defibrillation. Studies show that delay in achieving

defibrillation diminishes the chance of successful cardioversion. The only exceptions to this are trauma, near drowning and paediatrics when the primary cause of the arrest may be respiratory — in this situation, 1 minute of BLS should occur before going for help.

- Give two effective rescue breaths.
- Assess the patient for signs of Circulation.
- Check the carotid pulse for no more than 10 seconds.
- If there are no signs of a circulation, start chest compressions — if you are on your own, perform 15 compressions to two breaths.
- If there are two of you, perform five chest compressions to one breath.
- The breaths you deliver should make the mannequin chest visibly rise.
- Chest compressions should depress the sternum between 4 and 5 cm at a rate of 100 per minute.

BLOOD CULTURES

Examiners seem to prefer testing a student's ability to take blood cultures rather than pure venesection, as it further examines the student's ability to perform an invasive procedure using an aseptic technique.

- Introduce yourself to the patient and explain what you are about to do.
- Place the tourniquet around an appropriate arm and locate a suitable vein, preferably in the antecubital fossa.
- Clean the area of skin over the chosen vein. Preferably iodine should be used but if you are given steri-swabs ensure that you allow a minute for the alcohol to carry out its antibacterial effect.
- Wearing gloves, venesect at least 10 ml of blood from the vein using a syringe and a green needle. This procedure should not be performed via a pre-existing venflon.
- Release the tourniquet, place cotton wool over the venepuncture site and withdraw the blood-filled syringe and needle.
- Apply pressure to the cotton wool and offer the patient some tape or a plaster to put on the venepuncture site.
- You may then transfer the blood into two blood culture bottles.

- Clean the entrance ports of each blood culture bottle with iodine or separate steri-swabs.
- Change the green needle and pierce the port with the needle and syringe until at least 5 ml of blood has been transferred into the first culture bottle.
- Withdraw the needle and syringe.
- Change to a further new needle and repeat this process in the other blood culture bottle.
- Ensure that the blood culture bottles are labelled and bagged with the patient's request form.

The examiners will be awarding marks for:

- patient communication
- aseptic technique
- safety with regard to handling and disposing of potentially contaminated sharps.

DEMONSTRATING CORRECT INHALER TECHNIQUE

The first thing to do is to check the patient's prior knowledge about inhalers. Does the patient know anybody who has an inhaler? Has the patient ever seen an inhaler used before? Does the patient know what the inhaler is used for? Remember that β_2-agonist inhalers such as Ventolin are used for symptomatic relief ('the blue one is the reliever'). Steroid-based inhalers, on the other hand, are used more in a prophylactic sense ('the brown ones are the preventers').

We would then recommend explaining in words exactly what the technique involves — why it should be used and when it should be used. You should then adopt the following technique to demonstrate how to use the inhaler using a placebo device:

- Demonstrate the inhaler technique on yourself in real time.
- Repeat the above, broken down and explain each step as you go along.
- Repeat the above, but this time get the patient to do the explanation, prompting if necessary.
- Get the patient to do it at normal speed.

It may be necessary to repeat this process several times before some patients are able to get the hang of it. Always check that the patient understands why, when and how to use the inhaler at the end of the interview. Patients often find written literature, particularly with pictures and a simple diagram, helpful in understanding the procedure.

WRITING A DISCHARGE SUMMARY

You may be given a set of clinical notes and asked to write a brief summary to the patient's General Practitioner. We recommend that you use a structured format as set out in Figure 3.5.1. There is some

---

Hospital Discharge Summary

Date: Patient details: Consultant's name:
                          Name:
                          Address:
                          Hosp No: Admission dates:
                          Date of birth:

Diagnoses: 1)
                          2)
                          3)

Dear Doctor,

History:

Examination:

Investigations:

Treatment and progress:

Drugs on discharge:

Information given to the patient:

Follow-up arrangements:

Yours sincerely

HOUSE OFFICER

Fig. 3.5.1 Hospital discharge summary.

evidence that using a structured approach is the best way of communicating complex information. Try to keep to one side of paper — this will encourage you not to include too much unnecessary detail. Make sure your writing is legible.

RECTAL EXAMINATION

You will not be asked to perform a rectal examination on a patient during finals. You may, however, be asked to perform a rectal examination on a mannequin. Remember to treat the mannequin as if it were a real patient. Ask the mannequin for permission to perform a rectal examination ('examination of the back passage'). You should explain, in outline:

- why you want to do it
- that it may be uncomfortable but that it shouldn't hurt
- that it may be a bit embarrassing
- that it should only take 1–2 minutes.

Ask the examiner to act as a chaperone, especially if the mannequin is female. Then wash your hands, glove up, turn the patient into the left lateral position with knees pulled up towards the chest. Talk in a reassuring manner to the mannequin throughout. Apply lubricating jelly to the tip of the right index finger and apply gentle, sustained pressure to the anal sphincter with the lubricated digit. Once the finger is inside the rectum, carefully feel the rectal mucosa for any irregularities, by performing a gentle sweeping motion with the finger. If the patient is male, carefully examine the prostate. This whole procedure is best performed if you adopt a semi-crouching position.

It is important to visit your local clinical skills laboratory and practise your rectal examination there before you come to your finals. The common findings in final MB are:

- normal examination
- stool only
- rectal cancer
- prostatic cancer
- benign prostatic hypertrophy.

KEY QUESTIONS

Practical OSCE stations

We have described in some detail the commoner practical skills OSCEs. Here are a few less common questions for you to think about. All of these questions have been asked as an OSCE in Final MB within the last 3–4 years:

- Male catheterisation
- Writing a drug chart
- Writing 'TTOs' (drugs to take home)
- Drawing up and administering intravenous antibiotics
- Demonstrating to a patient how to perform and record a peak flow measurement
- Handwashing and aseptic technique
- Performing an ECG
- Blood pressure measurement
- Venflon/i.v. fluids.

Use the basic principles we have outlined to think about how you would approach these questions.

PART 4

ETHICS

Basic principles of an ethical decision
Specimen cases

4

Ethics

Over recent years there has been a greater emphasis on examining students' ability to discuss ethical dilemmas and formulate approaches to difficult ethical scenarios. This could occur as an additional question at any stage of the exam but is more likely to be presented as a discrete scenario to discuss with the examiner.

One of the difficulties with ethics is that there is often no 'correct' answer. You could ask ten experts in the field and they would all have different views on the subject. At the time of writing this edition, several major ethical issues are being debated in the House of Lords. This may result in changes in the law with regards to euthanasia/physician-assisted suicide, withdrawal of feeding and treatment of mentally incapacitated adults, to name but a few. We recommend you check the current legal standpoint on these areas in the weeks leading up to the exam. The BMA website has an excellent section on ethics.

So, if you get an ethical question, what do you need to do to pass? First and foremost, you must not do anything that may fail you! This includes:

- Demonstrating uncaring or unstable behaviour: 'I don't think smokers should be given vascular surgery. It's their own fault that they're in the mess they are in.'
- Demonstrating opinions that suggest you would be willing to break the law in clinical practice: 'I don't have a problem with overdosing terminal patients with morphine. They're going to die anyway.'
- Being unable to identify with opinions contrary to your own: 'No-one should have an abortion. It is unacceptable in all circumstances.'
- Being unaware of the basis upon which ethical decisions are made.

Your job is to demonstrate to the examiner that you have a sound appreciation of the basic principles upon which an ethical decision is made, and, with these principles in mind, discuss the main issues pertinent to the ethical dilemma. All the examiner really wants to see is that you are not going to do or say anything scary that may end up with you in court or in front of the General Medical Council.

BASIC PRINCIPLES OF AN ETHICAL DECISION

When approaching any ethical dilemma, it is always helpful to use these principles as a framework. It helps clarify the issues and demonstrate that you have looked at all the pertinent features.

The principles are:

- autonomy
- beneficence
- non-maleficence
- justice.

Autonomy

Autonomy is defined as 'the right of self-government'. In other words, patients of sound mind have the right to accept or decline the treatment offered. They have the right to make decisions regarding their health care and should be empowered to do so. Many ethical issues are concerned with patients who are unable to make their wishes known, who cannot use their autonomy. In this situation, the other principles will be more important in decision-making.

Example

Mrs Jones has been diagnosed with colon cancer and you recommend she be admitted to hospital for an operation. She states that she does not want an operation and understands that without one she may die. The ethical principle of autonomy dictates that you must respect her wishes. In fact, forcibly admitting her to hospital would constitute assault.

Even though we must respect a patient's autonomy, sometimes the law prevents us from doing so. A good example of this is physician-assisted suicide. A patient of sound mind may wish to have life ended but the law (as it stands) prevents a doctor from complying with the patient's wishes.

Beneficence

Beneficence is the act of doing good. In the medical situation, beneficence dictates that when we make a decision it should be done with the intention of *benefiting* the patient. Often we have to weigh this up against the harm that a decision may cause.

Example

Jimmy is a 4 year old diagnosed with leukaemia. He requires a bone marrow transplant and chemotherapy, which is likely to make him unwell. However, the intention is to cure him of this disease so that he can live a long and happy life. Beneficence would dictate that the proposed treatment is appropriate.

Non-maleficence

Maleficence is the act of doing something harmful. Non-maleficence is therefore the act of *not* doing something harmful. In medical situations non-maleficence is important in weighing up whether doing or not doing something will cause the patient harm. If we consider the above example of Jimmy and his leukaemia, non-maleficence could dictate we should not give him chemotherapy because it will make him unwell. However, not giving treatment would result in certain death and so non-maleficence would also argue that he should be treated.

Hmmm. Complicated, isn't it! It isn't really. We all know that Jimmy should be treated because even though the chemotherapy may be unpleasant, it is a necessary evil in order to cure his disease. So we see that the argument of beneficence comes into play.

Note. Whenever considering the pros and cons of a decision, beneficence and non-maleficence need to be weighed up together. Rarely can a decision be argued on the basis of just one of them. Both need to be considered.

Justice

This concerns what is legally and morally right in keeping with a person's religious and cultural beliefs. The bottom line is that you cannot make a decision that will result in breaking the law.

Example

Mrs Peters has advanced motor neurone disease. She knows that her condition is progressive and irreversible. She saw a friend from the MND support group die uncomfortably and is terrified that she will experience the same. She asks you to give her a lethal dose of sedative rather than continue this existence.

Regardless of what you argue regarding autonomy, beneficence and non-maleficence, none of these can overturn the fact that physician-assisted suicide is currently illegal in the UK. Therefore, justice dictates that you cannot give her a lethal injection.

Justice is also about fairness and may be used to balance arguments between autonomy and beneficence. It often provides a safeguard for staff and other patients.

Example

Miss Donovan is a 67-year-old with advanced breast cancer. She has lung, liver and bone metastases and is no longer receiving chemotherapy. She has been admitted with worsening breathlessness due to overwhelming infection and progressive lung disease. She is deteriorating despite antibiotics and her family want her admitted to the intensive care unit for ventilation. It is highly unlikely that this patient would benefit from ventilation and would almost certainly die on ITU. The ethical principle of justice compels us to consider fair use of finite resources: if she goes to ITU, someone who is more likely to benefit will not be able to.

SPECIMEN CASES

We have provided a few ethical dilemmas for you to consider. We have also included some commentary as to how to answer them. With each situation, we suggest you should first consider the four principles and then formulate an opinion. We have not put down the final opinion because this would reflect our own considered views and not yours!

Case 1

Mrs Jackson is dying of advanced cancer. She is in a side room, with her family present. She is unconscious and has a syringe driver, which contains diamorphine and midazolam. She is no longer taking anything orally.

What are the ethical issues regarding starting intravenous fluids?

Autonomy

Since she is unconscious and unable to communicate, she cannot make her wishes known. However, she may have made her wishes known on prior occasions in conversations or via an advance directive. You should make every effort to take into account her wishes when making a decision.

Beneficence

Intravenous fluids will prevent her from dehydrating. This may also be reassuring to the family members who often express concerns that their loved one may feel dry if she doesn't have fluids.

Non-maleficence

There are risks with starting intravenous fluids. In the terminal stages there is a greater likelihood of fluid overload, which will contribute to 'death rattle' and oedema. Cannulation can be uncomfortable, and may cause local phlebitis and infection.

Justice

Starting fluids is a medical intervention and legally doctors are not obliged to instigate a treatment which they feel is futile. Fluids are not going to alter the outcome and doctors may not feel they are appropriate.

Case 2

Mr Foley has advanced chronic obstructive pulmonary disease (COPD). He is on home oxygen and gets breathless on making a cup of tea. He is admitted with a chest infection and is being appropriately and actively treated. Despite this, he continues to deteriorate. Following review by the intensive care consultant, he is not considered a candidate for ventilation. One of the nurses asks you about his resuscitation status.

What are the ethical issues?

Autonomy

Assuming he is competent, he is able to make his wishes known. However, he may be confused due to hypoxia, hypercapnia, sepsis or exhaustion. If so, he will be unable to exercise his autonomy.

Beneficence

Cardiopulmonary resuscitation (CPR) will not offer any benefit to Mr Foley. Deciding against resuscitation will allow the team to prepare him for a peaceful death by concentrating on symptom control rather than aggressive invasive treatment. Sensitive discussion and involvement of the family will help minimise complicated bereavement.

Non-maleficence

CPR is highly unlikely to bring him back from an arrest. It may cause more injury such as broken ribs and hypoxic brain damage. If successfully resuscitated, he will still die but a few days later on a ventilator.

Justice

The only way this man will survive an arrest is by intubation and ventilation. He has already been assessed as not suitable for ITU and, if admitted now, he will prevent someone else who really needs a bed from being admitted to the ward.

It is unfair on the patient, staff and family to instigate futile treatments and legally doctors are not obliged to do so. However, if there has been a clinical decision not to resuscitate, asking Mr Foley's views may be unethical on the grounds of non-maleficence, as it may distress him to know that, despite wanting CPR, he would not get it. It highlights the importance of good communication skills and is covered in more detail in *Communication Skills for Final MB*.

Case 3

Mrs Jenkins is an 80-year-old woman presenting with obstructive jaundice. She almost certainly has cancer of the pancreas, but histology is awaited. Her granddaughter approaches you and asks that you do not tell her the diagnosis because 'She wouldn't be able to handle the news. It would be too much of a shock.'

What ethical issues need to be considered?

Autonomy

Mrs Jenkins is mentally competent and able to make her wishes known. If she wants to know the diagnosis, we must respect her autonomy in making this decision. Likewise, you can ask her what she wishes to know: some patients state they do not want to be told bad news. You are obliged to give her a choice.

Beneficence

Giving her the diagnosis will allow her to be informed in decision-making, e.g. chemotherapy or going home to die. Unless she has the facts she will be unable to do this.

Non-maleficence

If we collude with the granddaughter, it will eventually come out. Mrs Jenkins is likely to lose trust in those treating her and so it is beneficent to tell her the truth. Hence it may be harmful not to tell her.

Justice

Legally we have duty of care to the patient and, although we try to look after relatives as well, they are not our prime concern. If Mrs Jenkins wants to know the diagnosis we should tell her. From a fairness point of view, justice can argue that not telling her will make further treatment planning and care delivery difficult for the staff.

Case 4

Mr Roberts is a 62-year-old man with autoimmune liver disease. He is admitted with a torrential bleed from known oesophageal varices. On admission he states that he is a Jehovah's Witness and refuses to have any blood products. Without an urgent transfusion, he is likely to die.

What are the ethical issues?

Autonomy

So long as he understands the consequences of refusing transfusion we must respect his decision.

Beneficence

Blood transfusion would improve his physical health and save his life.

Non-maleficence

The consequences of forcing him to have a blood transfusion would be psychologically devastating.

Justice

Legally, if we forced him to have a transfusion it would constitute assault. Although this man's reasons for refusal are religious, we would have to respect his decision even if his reasons were illogical, irrational or non-existent.

PART 5

EVIDENCE-BASED MEDICINE

5

Evidence-based medicine

Evidence-based medicine (EBM) is becoming an increasingly important part of modern clinical medicine and you will be expected to understand the basic principles. This chapter explains the basic concepts of EBM that you are likely to be asked about.

WHAT IS EBM?

Evidence-based medicine is the integration of clinical expertise with the best available evidence in making clinical decisions about individual patients. Note that there are two key aspects to its successful application:

- clinical expertise
- application of best available evidence.

Only through clinical expertise (learnt at the bedside and from the rest of this book!) can doctors develop the skills needed to correctly identify clinical problems, thus enabling a relevant search for the best evidence. Clinical expertise is essential for the true practice of EBM.

Incorporating clinical expertise into your definition of EBM will help avoid trouble and negates the arguments that EBM is an attempt to usurp the traditional role of clinical medicine/teaching by the introduction of 'cookbook' medicine.

Best evidence is covered in the rest of this chapter.

The practice of EBM is an integral part of clinical governance. Clinical governance is topical and examiners may feel it is fair to ask questions about it. Clinical governance is a global approach to quality management within the health service. It is an attempt to bring together previous quality initiatives such as clinical audit, the *Patients' Charter* and clinical guidelines.

Two new institutions have been created by the UK government to help implement clinical governance. The National Institute for

Clinical Excellence (NICE) will produce evidence-based guidance for clinicians about difficult clinical issues (e.g. NICE has examined the role of β-interferon in the treatment of multiple sclerosis). The Commission for Health Improvement (CHI or CHImp) will focus on the *process* of delivering health care and how well institutions achieve this. For example, CHImp will examine a hospital trust's records on clinic waiting times for patients suspected of having cancer.

PRACTICAL EBM

There are five key components to practising EBM:

- converting clinical problems into answerable questions
- searching for and finding the best evidence to answer the questions
- critically appraising the evidence (also known as 'trashing papers')
- applying the evidence to our everyday practice
- auditing or evaluating our practice.

For example, on your first day as a doctor you see a 65-year-old man with a 4-hour history of ischaemic cardiac chest pain. There is nothing abnormal to find on examination, however an ECG shows ST-segment elevation in leads II, III and a VF, suggesting an acute inferior myocardial infarction (MI). Your registrar administers streptokinase and aspirin and on the ward round your consultant asks what evidence there is to support your registrar's action.

Answerable questions

Every day we are faced with clinical problems that we don't know the answers to. The most efficient way to find the answers is to convert these clinical dilemmas into answerable questions. These questions usually have four components (here, dealing with the example described above):

- *the patient or problem* — in a 65-year-old man with an uncomplicated acute MI (presenting within 4 hours of onset), what is the best treatment?
- *the intervention* — thrombolysis with streptokinase

- *the comparison intervention* — compared with standard therapy alone (i.e. in trials placebo)
- *the outcomes* — mortality reduction.

This question is probably very similar to most constructed in this situation. However, if you can get into the habit of using this format all the time, it makes things easier when dealing with more complicated situations.

Searching

Searches for evidence need to be thorough but efficient and computer databases (e.g. Medline) have helped greatly in achieving this. The best way to learn efficient searching is to be taught by your local medical librarian.

Critical appraisal

Critical appraisal is the art of finding the best evidence and discarding the rubbish. In this example, you would hopefully find trials comparing streptokinase/aspirin and placebo for the management of acute MI. The results from the trial may suggest that giving streptokinase is of benefit, but you have to decide if the trial methodology was sound enough to let you believe the conclusions. How you can achieve this is discussed later in the chapter.

Applying best evidence

Applying best evidence in a health care environment is not easy. Guidelines are one successful method for changing clinical practice. Guidelines should be evidence-based statements produced to assist clinicians in the management of clinical problems. Guidelines are only guides, however, and on occasion there are good clinical reasons not to follow them. In most hospitals there should be evidence-based guidelines for the management of acute MI.

Audit/evaluation

Audit or evaluation of practice is vital to ensure best evidence is implemented. Audit is a cyclical process in which current practice is evaluated (against set standards), any deficiencies are highlighted and as a result practice is changed. Practice should then again be observed, thus completing the cycle (Fig. 5.1).

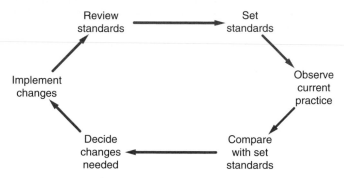

Fig. 5.1 The clinical audit cycle.

CRITICAL APPRAISAL: TYPES OF CLINICAL STUDIES

In order to be able to critically appraise, you will need to understand the basic methodologies and structures of different studies.

Cross-sectional study

This type of study is a survey designed to determine the prevalence/frequency of a disease (or other clinical characteristic) within a defined population at that point in time, e.g. measuring the blood pressure of all patients attending the diabetic clinic to find the prevalence of high blood pressure in this population (Fig. 5.2).

Cohort study

A cohort study is a prospective observational study used to investigate risk and risk factors. In other words, a group (cohort) of people exposed to a risk factor (e.g. asbestos) for a disease (e.g. respiratory cancer) followed for a period of time (usually many years). Comparisons between different groups (including a control group) can be made to determine the relationship between a risk factor and disease. For example, in a study of American asbestos insulators followed for 29 years, the *relative risk* for developing respiratory cancer (compared with controls) was 9.2 (Fig. 5.3). This means that respiratory cancer is over nine times more likely to occur in the exposed group than in the control group, and if the groups are matched for all other risk factors then we can infer that asbestos exposure is a risk factor for developing respiratory cancer.

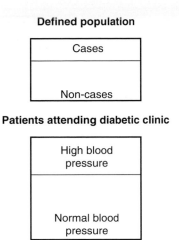

Fig. 5.2 Cross-sectional study.

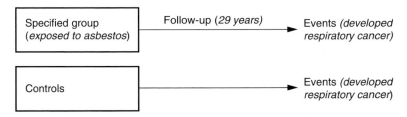

Fig. 5.3 Cohort study.

Case–control study

These are observational studies in which the characteristics of people with a disease (cases) are compared with the characteristics of a matched population (controls). A hypothesis is formulated, e.g. gastro-oesophageal reflux is a risk factor for adenocarcinoma of the oesophagus. Both groups' histories are examined to identify characteristics (including amount of reflux) and the results are expressed as an *odds ratio*. In this case (a large Swedish study), people with recurrent symptoms of reflux had an odds ratio of 7.7 for developing adenocarcinoma compared with the controls (the odds of developing adenocarcinoma is nearly eight times higher in patients with reflux than in those without reflux) (Fig. 5.4). To infer that the risk

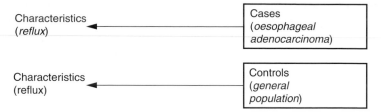

Fig. 5.4 Case–control study.

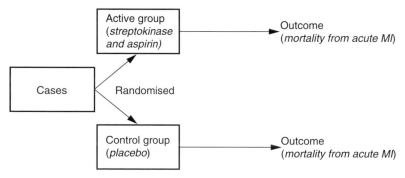

Fig. 5.5 Controlled trial.

factor identified is related to the disease in question, the cases and controls must have had similar exposure to other known risk factors (e.g. for oesophageal adenocarcinoma, smoking and alcohol intake).

Controlled trial

This is an interventional type of study. The treatment under investigation is given to one population of patients (active group) and their outcomes are compared with a similar population (control group) given another treatment or placebo. It is important that the two groups are otherwise treated identically. In the patient with the acute MI, the evidence for streptokinase and aspirin comes from ISIS-2 (International Study of Infarct Survival 2), in which patients with MI were allocated to one of four treatment arms: aspirin alone, streptokinase alone, aspirin and streptokinase together, or placebo (Fig. 5.5). There was significant benefit in receiving both streptokinase and aspirin (see below).

A randomised controlled trial (RCT) is a variation of the controlled trial and is regarded as the gold standard trial in the evaluation of new therapies. If you are given a paper to evaluate then there is a high chance it will be an RCT. A simple checklist can help you quickly decide if the trial is valid (i.e. if it has sound methodology enabling you to accept its results). Ask yourself the following questions:

- Were the patients randomised to treatment groups (this helps avoid bias in the study)?
- Were all the patients accounted for at the end of the study (it is amazing how many studies seem to 'lose' patients!)?
- Were patients *and* clinicians 'blind' to which treatment was being administered? (If this was the case then the study is said to be double-blinded. When only clinicians are aware of the treatment a patient is given then the trial is single-blinded.) Blinding helps to avoid placebo effects in patients and avoids clinicians' bias.
- Apart from the intervention under investigation, were all the groups treated equally (i.e. could any other factor have caused any difference in outcome)?
- Were the groups similar at the start of the trial (could the better outcome from the intervention be due to younger patients or patients with less severe disease in the active group compared with the control group)?

If the study meets the above criteria, the next thing to evaluate is the effectiveness (if any) of the treatment.

In ISIS-2 the group who received aspirin and streptokinase had a 5-week mortality rate (*experimental event rate*, EER) of 8% compared with 13.2% in the group given placebo (*control event rate*, CER).

This difference can be expressed in a number of ways.

The relative risk reduction (RRR) is the traditional method for expressing this difference (and the one often used by drug companies, as the figures look more impressive). The RRR is calculated as follows:

$$RRR = \frac{CER - EER}{CER} - \frac{13.2\% - 8\%}{13.2\%} = 42\%$$

i.e. streptokinase and aspirin reduced the chance of dying by 42%. However, the RRR ignores the underlying 'event rate' and fails to discriminate large benefits from small ones (see below).

The absolute risk reduction (ARR) is simply the absolute difference in outcomes between the groups. The ARR is calculated as follows:

Table 5.1				
Control event rate (CER)	Experimental event rate (EER)	Relative risk reduction (RRR)	Absolute risk reduction (ARR)	Numbers needed to treat (NNT)
100%	50%	50%	50%	2
10%	5%	50%	5%	20
1%	0.5%	50%	0.5%	200

$$ARR = CER - EER = 13.2\% - 8\% = 5.2\%$$

The ARR is a difficult concept to understand and an alternative way of expressing this, which is easier to visualise, is the concept of *numbers needed to treat* (NNT). The NNT is simply the inverse of the ARR:

$$NNT = \frac{1}{ARR} = \frac{1}{5.2\%} = \frac{1}{0.052} = 19.23 \approx 19$$

i.e. in acute myocardial infarction you need to treat approximately 19 people with streptokinase and aspirin to save one life at 5 weeks.

To demonstrate how data can be expressed in these different ways, imagine three hypothetical sets of results: the first set is of a condition which has 100% mortality reduced to 50% by a new treatment; the second shows a treatment that reduces mortality from 10 to 5%; and the third shows mortality reduction from 1 to 0.5%. The data are set out in Table 5.1. Note how hugely different NNTs and ARRs can have the same RRR.

Table 5.2 gives you a few examples of NNTs for some commonly used treatments. Note that when quoting NNT you should include a timescale which gives some idea of the duration of therapy needed to produce the outcomes.

Meta-analysis

Meta-analyses are studies in which all the valid evidence available for a particular subject, usually from RCTs, is statistically pooled. Increasing the number of subjects in the analysis in this way greatly increases the power (the probability of obtaining a true-positive

Table 5.2 NNTs for some common treatments

Condition	Intervention	Outcome prevented	Duration of follow-up	NNT
Acute MI	Streptokinase	Death	5 weeks	36
Acute MI	Aspirin	Death	5 weeks	42
Acute MI	Streptokinase and aspirin	Death	5 weeks 2 years	19 24
Diastolic BP 115–129 mmHg	Antihypertensives	Death, stroke or MI	1.5 years	3
Class IV congestive heart failure (CHF)	ACE inhibitor (enalapril)	Death	1 year	6
Class I or II CHF	ACE inhibitor (enalapril)	Death	1 year	100
Left main coronary artery stenosis	CABG	Death	2 years	6
Coronary artery disease	Simvastatin	Coronary death	5 years	29
Asymptomatic women aged 50–69	Breast examination & mammography	Death from breast cancer	9 years	1075

conclusion) of the study. The term 'systematic review' is often incorrectly used to mean meta-analysis. A systematic review is an overview of the subject, which may well include a meta-analysis, which strictly refers to the statistical process involved in pooling the data.

When deciding if a meta-analysis has been performed properly, there are two areas that deserve special scrutiny:

- How thorough a search for all relevant studies has there been? Historically, trials with positive results were more likely to be published than 'negative' trials. Thus, unless the search has been very thorough (including searching for unpublished trials) then there may be bias towards a positive result. The authors should state their vigorous search methods.
- The results of the pooled data can only be valid if the original studies they are derived from are of good quality. The methods

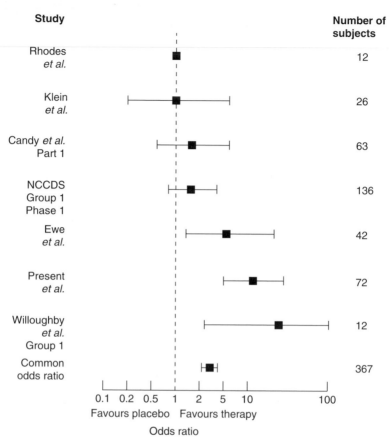

Fig. 5.6 The odds ratio for each study is represented by the filled squares, and the horizontal line passing through each square represents the 95% confidence interval. Odds ratios greater than 1 indicate a benefit from treatment compared with placebo. If the horizontal line crosses the vertical line representing an odds ratio of 1 then the result is not statistically significant (e.g. the study by Candy *et al.*). (Adapted from *Annals of Internal Medicine* 1995; 123(2): 132–142.)

section should explain how the quality of included studies was guaranteed and reassure that poor studies were rejected.

The results of meta-analysis are usually expressed as odds ratios (see earlier in chapter) and presented graphically as in Fig. 5.6, which shows the results of a meta-analysis of azathioprine or 6-mercaptopurine in active Crohn's disease.

SCREENING

It is worth knowing about screening for diseases for the final MB. Screening is the investigation (by history, examination or laboratory test) of asymptomatic people in order to identify an unrecognised disease or a risk factor for disease. Examples of screening include cervical smear testing for cervical cancer, mammography for breast cancer, and faecal occult blood testing for colorectal cancer.

Before widespread screening for a condition is introduced, the following criteria should be considered:

- Does the burden of disease warrant screening i.e. is the disease common and does it have a large impact (both economic and social) on society?
- Is there a good screening test? How sensitive and specific are the screening tests?
- Will the screening test be acceptable (i.e. not too invasive) and have low morbidity (remember screening involves investigating 'healthy' people)?
- If the screening identifies disease, is there an effective treatment that can be offered? If not, there is no point making an earlier diagnosis.
- Can the health system cope with the screening programme?
- Is the screening programme cost-effective?

Screening is controversial; two points worth remembering are as follows:

- Healthy people are being investigated and so any morbidity or even mortality associated with the screening test itself has to be seriously considered.
- The emotional, psychological and ethical aspects of subjecting healthy people to invasive and stressful medical investigations need to be considered.

Index

Page numbers in bold indicate main treatment of a subject/headings in the text.